HIV/AIDS

HIV/AIDS:
Loss, Grief, Challenge, and Hope

Mary O'Donnell, R.N., M.H.M.
Fort Lauderdale, Florida

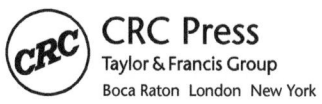

CRC Press
Taylor & Francis Group
Boca Raton London New York

CRC Press is an imprint of the
Taylor & Francis Group, an **informa** business

A TAYLOR & FRANCIS BOOK

HIV/AIDS: Loss, Grief, Challenge, and Hope

First published 1996 by Taylor & Francis.

Published 2022 by CRC Press
2385 NW Executive Center Drive, Suite 320, Boca Raton FL 33431

and by CRC Press
4 Park Square, Milton Park, Abingdon, Oxon, OX14 4RN

CRC Press is an imprint of Taylor & Francis Group, LLC

© 1996 Taylor & Francis Group, LLC

**Visit the Taylor & Francis Web site at
http://www.taylorandfrancis.com**

**and the CRC Press Web site at
http://www.crcpress.com**

A CIP catalog record for this book is available from the British Library.

Library of Congress Cataloging-in-Publication Data

O'Donnell, Mary (Mary Sharpe)
    HIV/AIDS : loss, grief, challenge, and hope / by Mary O'Donnell.
        p.   cm.
    Includes bibliographical references.

1. AIDS (Disease)—Patients—Care.   2. AIDS (Disease)—Psychological
aspects.   I. Title.
RC607.A26036   1996
362.1'969792—dc20   95-45406
                                                                              CIP

ISBN 13: 978-1-56032-329-7 (hbk)
ISBN 13: 978-1-56032-330-3 (pbk)

This book was set in Times Roman by Sandra F. Watts. The editors were Christine Williams and Kathleen P. Baker. Cover design by Michelle Fleitz. Printing and binding by Braun-Brumfield, Inc.

To Roger Galligan, November 1, 1948–September 23, 1992
Advocate, teacher, and dear friend

Contents

Acknowledgments

I am deeply grateful for the time, insight, and commitment that were shown to me by the HIV/AIDS team at the Children's Diagnostic Center and the staff at Broward House.

I thank all of the members of the HIV support group at the Broward Correctional Women's Institute for allowing me to be a part of their lives. I particularly acknowledge Elizabeth Vogt for her constant support and quiet leadership.

This book became a reality because of the initial and continuing encouragement of Ron Wilder and the friendship of B. J. Buntrock. Elaine Pirrone at Taylor & Francis has enthusiastically shepherded me through the process.

Guy, my beloved husband, made the dream come true. He typed, retyped, corrected, and cajoled with patience, humor, and persistence. I thank him from the bottom of my heart.

Preface

In 1984, I was privileged to meet a 23-year-old White gay male, Jonathan, whose face and torso were outrageously scarred and ravaged from Kaposi's sarcoma, a cancer virtually unknown in the United States and until the advent of AIDS thought to be peculiar to older men of Jewish extraction living on the coastline of the Mediterranean Sea.

Jonathan was witty, charming, rail thin, afraid, and in severe physical pain. The Kaposi's sarcoma had internalized, attacking the mucous membranes of his eyes, nose, mouth, and major organs.

At that time, not only was the general public terrified of this apparently new retrovirus, but the media carried many stories and pictures of professionals refusing to treat AIDS-infected people. Funeral directors outfitted themselves in protective gear that looked more appropriate for an odyssey in outer space than for readying individuals for their last earthly journey. Gay men found their jobs, homes, and lives jeopardized if there was so much as a hint that they might be HIV-infected.

Jonathan had not left his apartment in 6 weeks because he was afraid that if his landlord saw him, he and his lover would be thrown out on the streets. He was also fearful that his lover would lose his job as a waiter if Jonathan's disease became known, and the end result, homelessness, would inevitably occur. Their lives were further complicated by the fact that Jonathan was an illegal alien, and both of them were using the same Social Security number in the belief that at some time Jonathan would be able to qualify for Medicaid.

HIV/AIDS losses are often uniquely complex and strike at the very heart of individuals, life partners, families, extended families, tax bases, health care systems, and entire nations.

We are now in the second decade of HIV. If a cure were to be found today, individuals of all ages would still continue to be infected, and the majority would eventually develop signs and symptoms, followed by opportunistic infections and subsequent death.

At the same time, many who have reached deeply into their hearts and pockets are no longer among us to provide care, support, advocacy, and political leadership as they too were infected and have now died.

This book is for those professionals who are new to the field of HIV/AIDS. It is written from the perspective of the loss and grief attached to the diagnosis and progression of the infection and the challenge and opportunities that arise for the health professional to provide a continuum of responsive and positive care, thus encouraging the client, the family, lifetime partners, and friends to live their lives as well as possible.

The chapters address individual and support care needs from a practical intervention perspective intended to empower the client and caregivers. Subject matter ranges from an overview of what is currently happening worldwide in the transmission of HIV; the grief that is felt at the time of diagnosis; the needs of women and children; the complexity of legal issues; the bureaucratic jungle of Medicare, Medicaid, and Social Security; residential facilities, including women's prisons; the spiritual dimension, which is often neglected in our health care thinking; death, grief, bereavement, and survival; the recognition of one's own battle against fatigue syndrome with positive steps for stress management; and some observations as to where HIV is currently and where it appears to be going.

The book is reader friendly and offers helpful, nonjudgmental, practical guidelines to those working in the HIV/AIDS arena. HIV is no respecter of persons. Anyone can get it. As such, we must own it and recognize that people's needs, desires, and hopes are even more challenging when they know that their lives may be limited.

Throughout the book first names or pseudonyms are used, but each history is real. Many have now died. Without them, their love, their generosity of spirit, and their ability and desire to make a difference, this book would remain a niggling thought in the recesses of my mind. In their memory, I hope that the contents will make a difference to you.

Mary O'Donnell
Fort Lauderdale, Florida

1

HIV/AIDS: Past, Present, and Future

I had not thought that death had undone so many—T. S. Eliot, "The Waste Land"

Where did HIV/AIDS come from, where is it now, and where is it going? Is it different from other terminal diseases, and if so, why? Why has this tiny, mercurial, stubborn, and stealthy retrovirus affected so much of the world, wreaking havoc and chaos within families and countries?

As the virus continues its inexorable spread worldwide, it is critical that we learn the lessons that the past has taught us, analyze the present, and maximize our future resources as expediently as possible to prevent further spread and to humanely care for those already infected.

While the industrialized countries are struggling to find the most cost-effective method to provide adequate health care to their citizens, developing countries are frequently hard pressed to provide basic survival needs, let alone shoulder the enormous financial costs inherent with HIV/AIDS prophylactic intervention and continuing treatment. This is a challenge indeed!

THE PAST: THE UNITED STATES

Discovery of the Retrovirus

In 1981, physicians in the San Francisco Bay area of California began to see small numbers of gay men infected with an unusual protozoan parasite identified as *Pneumocystis carinii*; this infection became known as *Pneumocystic carinii* pneumonia. Other gay men were developing a rare neoplasm called Kaposi's sarcoma, whose lesions could cover the body externally and might also internalize to attack some or all of the major organs. Up until this time, Kaposi's sarcoma had been believed to occur only in elderly men of Jewish extraction who lived on the shoreline surrounding the Mediterranean. In Jewish men it did not internalize and was

1

most frequently seen as skin lesions between the knee and the ankle. Both the protozoan infection and the cancer appeared to be opportunistic as they only occurred in individuals whose immune system had been compromised by an unknown infection that caused massive destruction of the T4 lymphocytes.

Extensive research followed, particularly that by Luc Montagnier and his coworkers at the Pasteur Institute in France and by Robert Gallo and his colleagues at the National Institutes of Health (NIH) in Washington, D.C. By late 1983, it was generally believed that the cause of such enormous ebullient destruction of the white blood cell system was the variant of a minute, fragile, parasitic cancer-causing retrovirus identified as LAV (by the Pasteur Institute), HTLV-111 (by NIH), and ARV (by Jay Levy of the University of California).

By 1986, an international committee on nomenclature renamed the retrovirus *human immunodeficiency virus*, or HIV. *HIV-positive* (HIV+) refers to an individual whose blood tests positive for HIV antibodies and who is often asymptomatic but who becomes infectious shortly after transmission of the retrovirus. *Acquired immunodeficiency syndrome* (AIDS) is still the term used to describe the move from an asymptomatic stage to signs, symptoms, and opportunistic infections, and a person with AIDS is frequently referred to as a person with AIDS (PWA) or person living with AIDS. For consistency, PWA is used in this book. *HIV spectrum disease* rather than the term *HIV/AIDS* more accurately describes the range of years that may occur from the initial infection to its terminal and death stages.

In the early 1980s, my own experience was that individuals were diagnosed after the development of signs and symptoms, rapidly progressed into at least one opportunistic infection, and died within 6 months to a year after their diagnosis.

Political Attitudes

For years, federal and the majority of state, county, and local governments successfully ignored the possibility that this tiny retrovirus could spread into all populations, apparently hoping that it would remain in the gay or drug-injecting communities, traditionally areas politicians and society prefer to neglect or forget. Sadly, some states still manifest this "head-in-the-sand" and "it-will-go-away-if-we-ignore-it" approach. The consequences are being seen in the lack of prevention policy and the continuing spread of the retrovirus. This attitude forced the gay community to look after their own; and this they did, with love, dedication, money, education, outrage, outspokenness, and eventually with such political clout that government at all levels was forced to pay attention.

The Advocates

Individuals and organizations became verbal, astute, effective campaigners. They included Larry Kramer, Randy Shilts, the Gay Men's Health Crisis in New York City, the Whitman-Walker Clinic in Washington, D.C., the SHANTI project in San Francisco, the Health Crisis Network in Miami, and Center One in Ft. Lauderdale, to name but a few. Their voices screaming in the wilderness were to eventually produce a plethora of government-sponsored prevention, education, and treatment programs targeted at all levels of society. Funding is now available through the Ryan White Bill (created by the federal government in honor of the memory of young Ryan White who, in his early teens and infected with HIV, advocated for better understanding, care, and treatment), Medicare, Medicaid, and individual state-funded programs.

The private sector—spearheaded by the Robert Woods Johnson Foundation and followed by the American Foundation for AIDS Research, the National Community AIDS Partnership, the United States Conference of Mayors, and many, many other large and small sources—was to provide invaluable monies and cooperative ventures for research, prevention, care, and treatment when federal and state funds were abysmally lacking. Thankfully, they continue to do so today.

The Surgeon General

The one outstanding national figure during those barren years of minimal policy, prevention, and intervention strategies was the Surgeon General at that time, C. Everett Koop, who was outspoken, ethical, practical, and objective, and provided thoughtful leadership when no one else could or would. It was Dr. Koop who saw that an HIV/AIDS prevention pamphlet was sent to every household in the United States and released the Surgeon General's Report on AIDS in October 1986, thus commencing the task of bringing HIV into the open and into the political agenda.

The Gay Community

In the meantime, the gay–bisexual communities of large cities, particularly San Francisco, New York, and Miami, were decimated by the disease, which created thousands of mourners who continued to reach into their pockets and their hearts to help wherever it was needed. The United States should be forever grateful for the leadership that this group provided when it was so dismally lacking elsewhere.

During this time, talents and tax bases were lost that are irreplaceable for this generation. The population that was so heartbreakingly affected was largely young, White, middle to upper-middle class, earning excellent salaries, paying their taxes, and contributing unique skills and abilities, particularly in the world of the arts, literature, and entertainment.

An article in *Newsweek* (Ansen et al., 1993) called these unique men a lost generation and went on to list Michael Bennett, Rudolph Nureyev, Rock Hudson, Robert Mapplethorpe, Freddie Mercury, Perry Ellis, Tony Perkins, Liberace, Keith Haring, Denholm Elliot, Halston, and many others less famous but equally creative who had already died. As the *Newsweek* article so succinctly said, "a single death creates a cultural chain reaction" (p. 16).

As HIV has reached into other communities, so have come the diagnoses and deaths of other well-known figures such as Arthur Ashe and the infection of such superstars as Magic Johnson and Greg Louganis. One can only pray that preventive vaccines and medications effecting a cure will be found before hundreds of thousands more lives are lost.

THE PAST: THE WORLD

The Spread

The pandemic of HIV/AIDS is unprecedented in modern medical history, posing worldwide the most serious public health challenge imaginable. According to the 1992 World Health Organization's (WHO's) capsule summary on the pandemic, "extensive spread appears to have occurred in the late 1970's or early 1980's" (p. 3) By 1992, WHO estimated that between 9–11 million adults were HIV-infected and that approximately 1 million children had been born infected.

One of the reasons for the inexorable global spread of HIV/AIDS was the denial of many countries and individuals that it was a disease that would affect them; they preferred to perceive it as a disease peculiar to gay males, injecting drug users, or frequenters of prostitutes or as an African, American, or capitalist disease, according to the national view of the individual country. Thus, preventive education started late and is in a constant state of "catch up." When recognition finally occurred that this was "our" disease rather than "their" disease, panic was often the next response, resulting in fragmented and scattered preventive policies and strategies.

Sub-Saharan Africa

The predominant spread in sub-Saharan Africa was heterosexual and because of the tremendous weight loss associated with the wasting syndrome was often referred to as "slim" disease. Because of its mode of heterosexual transmission, children under 5 were particularly affected, often infected before birth and born into a home where both parents and other siblings were infected. Babies and young children grew up in households where their own survival was jeopardized and where one or both parents died prematurely.

Health budgets were stretched to the maximum as PWAs filled hospital beds and the demand for prevention, treatment, and care monies continued to escalate. As in so many other countries, there was often stigmatization of infected persons, causing isolation and abandonment, sometimes by close family members.

Tradition discouraged women from talking about sex or negotiating the issue of safer sex, within or outside marriage. Much of the population of sub-Saharan Africa lives in rural areas "where cultures and traditions still heavily determine family relations, and we need messages that are appropriate to this context to reach these women" (Made, 1994, p. 7). By late 1993, WHO's global program on AIDS estimated that the area had 7 million infected people. As a friend of mine who volunteers as an AIDS educator in Uganda asked, "How do you culturally replace a whole generation?"—a horrifying question for which an adequate answer seems impossible.

India

India is the world's second most populous country. Its past reaction to HIV/AIDS was often that of controversy, inaction, and denial. Infected blood donors, injecting drug users, the methods used for family planning, the exclusion of women from making their own medical decisions, migrant workers who may have unprotected same-sex relationships when they are away from home, and the selling of sex within family systems have all contributed to the continuing increase of HIV.

In respectable neighborhoods, women in posh houses sell sex from within "families" made up of a "father" or "uncle" (the broker), a "mother" or "aunty" (the madam) and four or five "daughters" with clients visiting during the evening or at night, usually with the "uncle" or "father." (Shreedar, 1994, p. 2)

Family planning concentrated on fertility control, not on protection against disease. Vasectomies, female sterilization, and intrauterine devices were effective against pregnancy, but not against the transmission of infections.

Culture, tradition, denial, and the lack of government leadership at a national and state level have led India into an increasing spiral of infection and prevention and treatment needs. In a recent HIV/AIDS prevention class in the United States, an Indian man who is a medical technologist working in the United States assured the group that only three people in his homeland were infected. He was distressed by and disbelieving of the WHO 1995 estimates that 1.6 million people in India may already be infected, although fewer than 500 cases of AIDS have been reported.

Central and Eastern Europe

For years, many Central and Eastern European countries regarded AIDS as a phenomenon of the West. These countries had well-defended and more or less impenetrable borders, enabling them to establish a *cordon sanitaire* of mandatory HIV-antibody testing for foreigners and nationals returning from the West. Infected nationals were allowed to return but were subjected to strict state monitoring (Hendricks & Krickler, 1991).

When the barriers of communism were breached and destroyed in 1989, so came huge changes in social structures, including the ability to travel freely, increasing tourism, worsening economic conditions for some, more social freedom for others, an independent media, more prostitution and street drug use, and changing political values and policies. How these changes will affect the spread of HIV remains to be seen.

Western Europe

HIV was first identified in the late 1970s and 1980s in large urban areas. The people most affected at that time were bisexual or gay men and injecting drug users. AIDS became one of the leading causes of death in young men aged 20–40 years, although in more recent years there has appeared to be a slow decline in the spread in the bisexual and homosexual community and an increase in heterosexual populations.

Western Europe politically and aggressively used the media through pamphlets, billboard campaigns, subway advertising, and public restrooms to provide specific information on how to prevent the spread of HIV. Advertisements used words and pictures that were crisp, graphic, and explicit, unlike their counterparts in the United

States. Condoms became available in airports, railway, and port terminals, and everyone was exhorted to protect themselves.

Some European countries had already legitimized street drugs and needle-exchange programs, which may have reduced some of the spread. Mirroring the United States's experience, many of the early strategies and interventions were developed by the population most affected, the gay male community, particularly the Terrence Higgins Trust in London, England, which is now one of the largest multicommunity and multiservice AIDS organizations in Europe. In 1983, the trust was established by friends of Terrence Higgins, one of the first people in Britain to die from AIDS. Since then it has committed itself to the needs of people with HIV/AIDS nationally and internationally.

Western Europe's HIV-infected population numbered 50,000 as of late 1993 and is growing.

Latin America and the Caribbean

An extensive spread of HIV began in the early 1980s in bisexual and gay men and in injecting drug users in large cities. Since the mid-1980s, sexual transmission between men and women has steadily increased and may now be the predominant cause of the spread between bisexual men and their female partners and female sex workers and their male clients.

Spread also occurred in those countries in which married women have only one sexual partner, their husband. Because the societal structure frequently sanctions relationships outside the marriage for men and condom use is considered unmasculine, husbands are vulnerable to contracting the virus and subsequently infecting their unknowing, unsuspecting spouses.

Infection rates among pregnant women in Brazil and the Caribbean are increasing, which will heighten the infection rate in newborn babies. Many countries of the region have suffered from political unrest, uncontrollable inflation, guerilla warfare, refugees from neighboring countries, social unrest, and poverty.

Monies for HIV/AIDS prevention, care, and treatment are frequently hard to come by and must compete with general health care funding. An increasing number of AIDS organizations are developing, which is encouraging. They will need continuing internal and external support if they are to be effective.

South and Southeast Asia

The extensive spread of HIV started in the mid-1980s, primarily through injecting drug use and sex with heterosexual partners. Heterosexual spread has advanced rapidly, particularly among those with multiple sex partners (WHO, 1992).

Countries such as Cambodia have widespread prostitution, ignorance, and high-risk behavior. Accompanying this may be poverty, the perception of women as second-class citizens, and weak economies. Blood donors are rarely screened, and hospitals and clinics may not effectively sterilize needles for regular medical injection use.

Other countries such as Korea have not seen a high HIV incidence so far. Indeed, Korea is in somewhat of a "catch-22" situation. The outside world sees it as a rich country, so international agencies will not fund either government or nongovernment HIV programs. Internally, there is little government funding and support for prevention; there is reticence to discuss sexual behaviors and attitudes, and the future for the spread of HIV is uncertain.

Although its first documented case of AIDS was in 1984, Japan still does not acknowledge its HIV problem. Health workers are resistant to caring for infected persons, and "the doors of most Japanese hospitals remain firmly shut to HIV and AIDS, and thousands of people with HIV are hidden from society under a blanket of fear and prejudice" (Bourke, 1995, p. 1). The present estimate of people infected varies from 3,166 to 20,000. Whether attitudes, behaviors, and care and treatment will change is impossible to predict.

The entire region of South and Southeast Asia is geographically large and diverse, with the majority of its people concentrated in large, overcrowded metropolitan cities and the remainder scattered throughout the rural areas. What the future will bring is dependent on the commitment of the governments concerned, AIDS organizations, and funding agencies to provide accurate and culturally appropriate prevention information and to institute humane treatment and care.

China

Very little is known about the past decade and China's HIV experience. What is known is that since China has welcomed more foreign trade and foreign visitors, the sex trade has increased and now has around 1 million sex workers. There may be 2.5 million drug users who mostly use heroin. Sexually transmitted diseases (STDs) are increasing, and it is assumed that HIV is as well.

Islamic Countries

There are now 1 billion Muslims throughout the world. Many are affluent and travel extensively. Information regarding AIDS in Muslim countries is not readily available. Islamic countries range from fundamentalism to liberalism and have a broad range of language and cultural diversities.

According to Mohammed Hanif (1995), many Muslims "believe that Islamic values provide a degree of protection against HIV" (p. 7). In Saudi Arabia, the law "requires women to cover themselves, the electronic and print media are strictly censored, drug pushers are beheaded publicly, there is a complete ban on all intoxicants and the word sex is absent from the public vocabulary" (p. 6). The taboos that surround prostitution, homosexuality, and extramarital sex and the stigma surrounding HIV have made it difficult for people to seek information and education. Statistics for the principal Islamic countries are not wholly reliable, but WHO has estimated that at least 100,000 cases have occurred in the Middle East and North Africa.

Many Muslim countries have begun to accept the presence of the disease. An increasing number of educational programs ranging from public seminars, posters, billboard campaigns, and radio and television messages are occurring. There is still much to be done, but a positive stance does appear to be happening in some locations.

SUMMARY OF THE PAST

In 1981, a new syndrome that became known as AIDS was first recognized among homosexual men by physicians in California. The same syndrome was seen in urban areas in Australasia and Western Europe. In 1982, the syndrome became apparent in sub-Saharan Africa among both men and women, and its spread throughout the world was occurring.

The first documented case of HIV dates back to 1959 and was found in a sailor from Manchester, England. After his death from unknown causes, his bodily tissue was taken and stored. When the tissue was tested years later, the AIDS virus was identified in it.

Researchers discovered that HIV/AIDS destroyed the cells known as CD4s, which are critical factors in maintaining a healthy immune system. Lack of CD4 cells prevents the body from defending itself against bacteria. The spread of HIV occurs by means of sharing infected human bodily fluids through unprotected sexual intercourse, infected injecting-drug users sharing needles, infected blood or tissue donors, transmission from an infected mother to her unborn child, and more rarely through human breast milk.

In 1987 the first drug used to fight HIV, an antiretroviral medication called zidovudine (AZT) was licensed by the Federal Drug Administration. Various research studies on AZT have found its use to be limited. Although it may prolong life, it cannot save people from eventual death and it does not delay the onset of AIDS for HIV-infected people who take it when they have no signs and symptoms.

By 1992, the number of AIDS deaths worldwide had reached 500,000 (Brown, 1995). Most countries were reporting cases of HIV/AIDS, more and more women and children were becoming infected, and the need for effective preventive measures and efficient treatments and care became more and more of a challenge. A wonderful breakthrough was reported at the beginning of 1994 when trials showed that the administration of AZT to infected mothers during their pregnancies cut the mother–child transmission rate by two thirds.

HIV/AIDS has struck down men and women in their most productive years and, unlike other terminal diseases, has affected and infected entire family systems. It is a social, economic, and spiritual catastrophe whose size is still unknown.

Is all lost? No, not if governments, local officials, educators, counselors, friends, advocates, administrators, philanthropists, and public and private businesses band together to develop public policies and strategies for education, prevention, intervention, treatment, and care.

THE PRESENT AND FUTURE CHALLENGE

The West

By March 1995,

the World Health Organization's Global Program on AIDS (GPA) stated that cumulative reported cases of AIDS in the world had reached 1,025,073—a 20% increase since

January 1994. The GPA estimates that 4.5 million cases of AIDS have actually occurred worldwide. Some 19.5 million people are reported to have been infected with HIV since the pandemic began, including 1.5 million children. ("WHO Figures," 1995, p. 4)

Enormous amounts of money are being poured into research by many different countries in many different areas of the world. Research has already led to a better understanding of the cause and effect of the retrovirus. Early detection, improved monitoring, and more effective treatment has changed the retrovirus into a manageable disease if individuals have access to skilled medical care and good support systems. Indeed, many of us in the United States have HIV-positive friends who have lived, and lived well, for 11 to 15 years without developing any signs, symptoms, or opportunistic infections. Although the majority of people infected in the West continue to be gay and bisexual men, in some areas these figures are beginning to plateau and, indeed, to decrease, particularly in the older gay population. Current predictions project that the rate of transmission through heterosexual contact will eventually be greater than that through gay and bisexual contact. Conversely, young gay or bisexual males, adolescents, and women and young children are showing a marked increase in HIV/AIDS. African American women of childbearing age are at particular risk and have a high transmission rate caused by their own injecting drug use or, more commonly, through heterosexual contact with an injecting-drug-using infected man.

HIV disease is first and foremost a disease of behavior, and often those behaviors are cloaked in taboos, denial, compromise, and powerlessness. The challenge is complex and strikes at the very framework of societal mores, ethics, economics, beliefs, and value systems. However, there is still much that can be done if there is desire, commitment, and action.

ACTION PLAN

We must

- recognize that current HIV health monies for research, education, prevention, and treatment are inadequate. This becomes a particular challenge when health care in the industrialized world is undergoing a major political and economic shift in interpretation and delivery. The rich will continue to be able to afford excellent care, but the middle class is already scrambling for adequate health care coverage in a marketplace that is becoming increasingly more difficult.
- recognize the needs of the large number of infants and young children, both infected and noninfected, who will lose, at the very least, their mothers and whose survival needs will depend on grandparents, other relatives, foster parents, and the state. In the United States alone, current predictions are that there will be between 72,000 and 125,000 children and teenagers orphaned by the year 2000 (Levine & Stein, 1994).
- educate teenagers who traditionally believe that they are invincible and immortal, who already have a high rate of STDs, and to whom monogamy often means one relationship at a time for a short time.
- identify, inform, and educate poor and traditionally underserved people, par-

ticularly women, to whom putting a meal on the table may be far more important than an HIV+ status.

- acknowledge prisoners who may die alone, with inadequate medical treatment, and who have long since ceased to be a threat to society.
- boldly intervene with runaway teenagers and homeless people who may be forced into prostitution and unsafe practices to provide themselves with basic survival needs.
- help develop self-esteem, negotiating skills, and sexual responsibility in mar-ried and single women whose spouses or lovers have affairs.
- reinforce the fact that condom use does not encourage promiscuity but does promote safer sex and saves lives.
- acknowledge that clean needles and needle-exchange programs in the injecting-drug-using culture do save lives.
- encourage nursing homes and adult day care centers to care for infected indi-viduals.
- offer health care professionals more and more HIV/AIDS education, particularly in areas related to loss, grief, bereavement, burnout, and their own health care.
- support a political agenda that aggressively encourages research into vaccines, prophylactic treatments, and curative and inexpensive pharmaceuticals.
- increase research treatment methodologies for women and children.
- support political agendas that penalize discrimination, protect confidentiality, adequately fund care and treatment, stimulate public awareness, and use adver-tising monies to realistically advertise condom use and clean needles because the message of abstinence is not enough.

The West is fortunate to have economies and research and treatment facilities that support people living with HIV/AIDS. There is still an enormous amount left to do before there is a cure, and as we move toward the year 2000 we have to remain vigilant and not allow the issues of HIV spectrum disease to fall from the media or public attention.

THE WORLD

Much of the rest of the world does not and will not have these benefits. The challenge for many countries becomes monumental when seen against the back-drop of rapidly changing states of nations, borders, political and economic infra-structures, heightened unemployment, mass migrations, and civil wars. However, HIV/AIDS cannot be ignored, and neither can it be seen as someone else's prob-lem, because it is not going to go away.

TACKLING THE PROBLEM

To tackle the problem, there needs to be

- pooling and sharing of knowledge and resources between developed and devel-oping countries.
- educational programs that fit the target audience in language, cultural sensitiv-

ity, accuracy, and repetitiveness and experimental and prescription drugs available to countries at a cost that is not prohibitive.

- good hygienic techniques available through cheap and easy access to soap, water, latex gloves, masks, and gowns.
- change in condoning women as second-class, disenfranchised human beings and teaching choices, empowerment, condom use, the art of negotiation, and self-esteem.
- acceptance of teenage gay boys and men so that they can feel comfortable about their sexuality rather than making it a disgraceful closeted event.
- a reduction of poverty, which all too often creates risky behavior.
- early diagnosis and treatment, which traditionally does not correlate with little education and low income.
- trained physicians to treat people who are infected; clean collection systems to ensure safer blood, plasma, and tissue supplies; and informed consent for those being tested for HIV.
- confidential and inexpensive HIV testing and counseling and early diagnosis and treatment of STDs.
- improved care for children, both physical and emotional.
- cessation of foreign trade to those countries that knowingly condone the sale of children of both sexes into the sex trade.
- more research into alternative treatments and traditional plant-based medicines.
- encouragement of sexual abstinence in teenagers.
- adoption and implementation of national nondiscriminatory AIDS policies.
- adoption of AIDS policies in the workplace.
- improvement in the distribution of funds and resources.
- institution of preventive education and regular medical care to sex workers of both sexes.
- trained counselors and lay people to facilitate support groups for those who are affected before and after death has occurred.
- aggressive preventive child abuse programs, particularly for the homeless; utilization of those resources and skills that volunteers so often offer and that can be found in community after community.
- the appointment of the affected community, including women and adolescents, to national policy committees.
- the participation of students, parents, teachers, and churches in the planning of school curricula for HIV/AIDS education.
- trained health care workers to provide care in the home.
- support for foster parents and elderly persons who have lost their own children and are now caring for their children's children.

The list goes on and on. It is to be hoped that our compassion and caring will keep step with this retrovirus as it continues its own progression.

CONCLUSION

HIV/AIDS is not going to go away in the near future. Since HIV/AIDS was first recognized in 1981, identified in 1983, and confirmed as being the almost definite cause of AIDS in 1984, it has continued to spread worldwide and is now pandemic. During this period progress has occurred. More is known about the transmission and cause of the disease, medications continue to be researched, 5% of the HIV population worldwide have not become symptomatic, and treating pregnant mothers with AZT has cut the risk of infection to their unborn babies by two thirds. Opportunistic infections can be aggressively treated with antibiotics and fungicides. What is still not known is how the virus actually destroys the immune system, if some strains of HIV are weaker than others, why there are those who have unprotected sex with infected partners and do not become infected themselves, and when there will be an effective vaccine against HIV.

Although most wealthy countries have the benefit of early diagnosis and treatment, use of high-priced drugs, and extensive health care and voluntary support systems, much of the remainder of the world is excluded because such resources are economically impossible.

The challenge is huge. We must listen to those infected and affected by HIV. More than anyone, they know what is needed and where it is needed, and they often have very sound ideas on how to implement these needs. We must strive to use our own particular and unique talents to educate sensitively, provide care with hope and without discrimination, to encourage research, and to provide loving shelter for the orphans and support for those who mourn. Individual commitment and caring make an enormous difference, but if we are to be successful in the fight against HIV/AIDS, then everyone has to participate.

REFERENCES

Ansen, D., Ames, K., Doote, D., Kroll, J., Kuflik, A., & Plagens, P. (1993, January 18). A lost generation. *Newsweek*, 16–20.
Bourke, P. (1995). Japan's climate of mistrust. *WorldAIDS, 38*, 1.
Brown, P. (1995). HIV: The story so far. *WorldAIDS, 37*, 5–9.
Eliot, T. S. (1992). The waste land. In *The waste land and other poems*. Buccaneer Books.
Hanif, M. (1995). AIDS and Islam. *WorldAIDS, 38*, 6–10.
Hendricks, A., & Krickler, K. (1991). *WorldAIDS, 15*, 3–15.
Levine, C., & Stein, G. L. (1994). *Orphans of the HIV epidemic*. New York: The Orphan Project.
Made, P. (1994). The way forward. *WorldAIDS, 36*, 7.
Shreedar, J. (1994). Behind closed doors. *WorldAIDS, 36*, 2.
WHO figures. (1995). *WorldAIDS, 38*, 4.
World Health Organization. (1992). *Current & future dimensions of the HIV/AIDS pandemic*. Geneva, Switzerland: Author.
World Health Organization. (1993). *The HIV/AIDS pandemic: 1993 overview*. Geneva, Switzerland: Author.

2

Anticipatory Grief:
The Crisis and the Challenge

Everything that limits us we have to put aside.
—Richard Bach, *Jonathan Livingston Seagull*

AIDS touches the very core of our emotional selves, whether we are infected or affected, interested or disinterested, or convinced that this disease cannot possibly happen to us. AIDS triggers intense reactions and responses, including denial, rage, stigma, sorrow, anxiety, depression, deprivation, helplessness, hopelessness, withdrawal, panic, guilt, suicidal thoughts, and the very real fear of a debilitating illness and subsequent death.

Unlike other terminal diseases that generally present themselves when people are older, usually attacking only one family member, HIV is a disease seen most often among young men and women aged 20–45, in the prime of their lives. Again, unlike the majority of other terminal diseases, family members, life partners, primary caregivers, and friends may also be infected. All the traditional support systems may therefore become very fragile or disappear entirely.

The mental health professional is indeed challenged to find appropriate choices and answers for the many complex issues that an HIV/AIDS diagnosis causes.

This chapter seeks to identify the questions and process associated with HIV/AIDS from transmission to possible death, the probability of anticipatory grief, the decisions that sooner or later have to be made, and suggestions for decision making and intervention that will encourage positive outcomes and help alleviate sorrow. The approach is generic and can be used by health professionals regardless of their ethnicity, gender, national background, cultural values, or belief systems. Do remember that whatever the reason for one's own involvement in this complex sphere, it needs long-term commitment, generosity of heart, a nonjudgmental attitude, and recognition that your best has to be good enough and that some issues are not always resolvable.

To protect oneself and to inform and support others, it is essential to know the ways in which HIV is and is not transmitted. Never has a retrovirus had more myths and fears associated with how it is spread than tiny, fragile, destructive HIV, so let us destroy the myths!

MODES OF TRANSMISSION

HIV is spread by the commingling of infected bodily fluids through anal, vaginal, and, rarely, oral sexual intercourse; sharing contaminated "dirty" needles and syringes from an injecting-drug-using infected person; contaminated sharp instruments such as needles, scissors, or cutting blades that cause punctures or wounds that break the skin; splashes of infected blood into mucosal membranes; and infected donated blood, plasma, tissue, or organs. It may also be passed from an infected mother to her child before or during birth or from breast milk after birth. Remember that outside the human body, HIV is very fragile and easily destroyed by wiping up spills of contaminated blood with household bleach or household detergents.

Now that you know how HIV is spread, let us look at how it is not spread. HIV is not spread by handshakes; coughs and sneezes; sweat or tears; food; mosquitoes or other insect bites; toilet seats; telephones or computers; straws, spoons, or cups; drinking fountains; or hugs and on-the-cheek kisses (Centers for Disease and Prevention, 1993).

Although it is easy to list how HIV is not spread, it is really important to remember that people, including health professionals, are tremendously scared by the possibility of exposure. Helping to work through those fears is essential if good care and support are to be provided. The easiest ways to do this are by confronting and discussing fears; providing supportive, easy-to-read pamphlets such as the Health and Rehabilitative Services (1990) booklet titled *About Living with HIV*; explaining and providing protective equipment if the person with AIDS (PWA) has copious bloody drainage; and demonstrating one's own lack of fear by touching and hugging. PWAs invariably have remarkable insight into other people's fears because they easily recognize all the nonverbal negative communication that may and does occur.

The following story demonstrates how difficult coping becomes when one feels isolated and rejected. Some years ago after an HIV information session, we made a circle and gave each other a huge group hug. An older man, new to the meeting, started to cry and ran out of the room. I hurried after him and he told me, between heart-wrenching sobs, that since his diagnosis 9 months earlier no one had touched him. People should never have to live that way. Addressing and reducing fear is vital for good interaction and healthy lifestyles.

The health professional must be aware that grieving almost always occurs when a diagnosis of HIV is given to the client. This is by no means unique to HIV and usually happens when any potentially life-threatening diagnosis is made. The difference is that with HIV the ramifications are often complex and affect many other people. This process is called *anticipatory grief*.

ANTICIPATORY GRIEF

Feelings of loss do not start as death occurs; rather, they begin when the diagnosis is first made, when the individual and surrounding family members and significant others are thrown into an extraordinary state of anguish in which all emotional energy is harnessed to the diagnosis and prognosis. Feelings of loss may be expressed by anger, guilt, withdrawal, frustration, betrayal, denial, shock, and threatening behaviors (Hinton, 1972).

Anticipatory grief is usually manifested in some shape or form by everyone who is diagnosed as HIV-positive (HIV+) and by those who love them. To be helpful, the counselor must remember that grief intervention must be practical as well as psychological. Grief issues surrounding the diagnosis may also include very real fears of losing one's job and therefore status, self-esteem, financial solvency, health insurance, and ultimately the basic survival needs of transportation, nourishment, clothing, and shelter. The HIV+ status may also include the loss of family or significant others. It is not easy, for instance, to telephone Mom and say "Hi, I'm gay/an injecting-drug user/sexually active and I also have AIDS." Mom (who seems to be the familial figure most frequently contacted), if any of this is a surprise and all too often it will be, is going to have to deal with her own expectations and loss issues and then intervene with Dad and the rest of the family. Sometimes this can prove to be the most binding, growing, and loving experience the family has ever experienced, but others may not survive it well and will deliberately separate themselves from the infected individual. Significant others may feel unable to cope and may choose to leave the relationship for a variety of reasons such as fear of losing their own good health, perceived financial loss, an inability to change roles, feelings of spiritual isolation, altered expectations, and the probability of an increasing burden over months or years. Fortunately, these problems seem to be more the exception than the rule.

The process of anticipatory grief is as hard to define as is the course of HIV spectrum disease. It is now agreed that with early medical and psychosocial intervention people can often live healthily for many months and, indeed, many years. Grieving becomes an event of the past, life is lived fully, and often individuals become convinced that they will lick this disease—and they may very well be right!

However, the majority will eventually develop signs and symptoms that at some time will be followed by one of several opportunistic infections. Anticipatory grief will almost certainly reoccur. This is the time when clients will recognize the full meaning of their life-limiting illness and may become exceedingly depressed and anxious. This is an opportunity for the health care professional to help clients to focus on their immediate needs and goals, for instance, is work becoming difficult because of fatigue and infections and is this when financial aid should be sought from federal, state, or local funding agencies; if financial support is necessary, will it be enough to pay for the basic survival needs of shelter, food, transportation, utilities, and medical expenses; if the person lives alone is there an adequate support system to help; is there unfinished business with anyone and can there be resolution; is there a need to identify and legally assign adoptive parents or for a living will, personal power of attorney, or a health care surrogate; or are there dreams that can still be accomplished, relatives and friends to see, letters to be written, or decisions to be made? Resolution of the individual's issues invariably brings feelings of accomplishment and relief and the ability to continue living with a huge decrease in anxiety.

Anticipatory grief manifests the expectation of loss before its actual occurrence. It is not limited to the affected person and family, but ripples out in a huge circle to encompass all those who are in any way associated with the individual.

Recognizing anticipatory grief and finding positive interventions will immeasurably assist clients to empower themselves and develop positive coping strategies. Among other things, it will also help them to identify risky behaviors that, if not changed, may further jeopardize their health and well-being.

RISKY BEHAVIORS

One of the main reasons that HIV continues its remorseless spread is that people just do not believe the preventive educational messages. This is particularly true of teenagers, whose most endearing and frustrating quality is that of absolute trust in their own invincibility and immortality. Unfortunately, that trust could be the death of them, and we need to provide ongoing factual information that is conveyed in a language and style to which they can relate.

Assessing and knowing our own risk factors is essential if we are to understand the risk factors of our clients. The 1993 Surgeon General's report (Centers for Disease Control and Prevention, 1993) to the American public suggests that if we can answer yes to any of the following questions, any one of us could be at risk for HIV infection and other sexually transmitted diseases (STDs).

1. Have you ever had unprotected sex (anal, vaginal, or oral) with a man or woman who you knew was infected with HIV? injects or has injected drugs? shared needles with someone who was infected? had sex with someone who shared needles? had multiple sexual partners? was someone you normally wouldn't have sex with?
2. Have you used needles or syringes that were used by anyone other than you?
3. Have you ever given or received sex for drugs or money?
4. Did you or any of your sex partners receive treatment for hemophilia between 1978 through 1985? have a blood transfusion or organ transplant between 1978 through 1985?

Just looking through the list is a reminder that many unsuspecting people may have inadvertently put themselves at risk, particularly during the fast-paced sexual revolution of the past 25 years. Once we understand what the risks are, it becomes easier to educate our clients about safer behaviors and healthier lifestyles. It is essential to remember that the only absolutely safe behaviors are no sex and no exchange of bodily fluids.

Safer behaviors include

- abstinence—absolutely, positively no sex
- monogamy, which means one uninfected partner forever—no other sexual relationships
- protected anal, vaginal, and oral sex—wearing a latex condom every time however much you think you know the other person
- discontinuing the use of injecting or any mind-altering drugs; using clean needles

and syringes every time and refusing to share drug paraphernalia ("works") with others, if stopping drug use is impossible
- decreasing alcohol intake
- health professionals following universal precautions where all clients are treated as if they may have an infectious disease
- living a healthy lifestyle such as eating nutritious food, exercising at least three times a week, and getting plenty of rest
- practicing good personal hygiene, particularly when washing hands; teaching small children when and how to wash their hands, how germs are spread, and how to keep cuts clean and covered
- regular physical examinations
- enrollment in a drug or alcohol rehabilitation program and developing healthy support systems

Now that risky, safe, and safer behaviors are identified, the health professional needs to have a clear understanding of what is meant by HIV testing.

HIV TESTING: WHY, WHEN, AND HOW

People choose to be tested for HIV antibodies for a variety of reasons, including previous risky lifestyles; persistent unexplained undiagnosed signs and symptoms; an infected partner; receiving donated blood or organs before 1985; contracting other STDs since 1975; a diagnosis of tuberculosis or hepatitis B or C; and donating blood, sperm, or organs. People may choose not to be tested because they are terrified of the possible consequences, would rather not know, do not believe they could be positive, perceive a positive result as a death sentence, or do not have access to medical services.

Deciding when to be tested is frequently surrounded by anguish, ambivalence, and dread. The counselor's task is to assist clients to come to this decision in their own time and to address the consequences of a positive result with their clients before testing. An example is a participant in an HIV bereavement support group who was terrified of being tested. The group encouraged him to take the test. When he said yes, three of them accompanied him to his physician's office. The results came back as positive. He had suspected this outcome but was nevertheless devastated. Ten days later he became extremely ill and was hospitalized with *Pneumocystis carinii* pneumonia. He eventually recovered and lived very well for another 4 years. Before his diagnosis he had not manifested a single symptom. Was the opportunistic infection a coincidence or an outcome of depression and despair following the test results? It will never be known.

QUESTIONS A CLIENT MAY ASK

Where Is the Test Done?

At Public Health departments, STD clinics, medical facilities, and physicians' offices. The counselor should ask the client whether there is a possibility that friends, relatives, or acquaintances may be at an STD or primary health clinic if the testing is done there, whether the client may be seen, recognized and questioned; and if this is OK?

How Much Does the Test Cost?

Public health clinics charge on a sliding scale from approximately $20 to zero. No one is turned away because of their inability to pay. Private physicians' fees are usually higher.

How Should It Be Paid?

Any way. Clients should consider that if it is claimed on a health insurance policy it will inform the insurer of both the testing and the HIV status.

Is It Confidential or Anonymous?

Confidential testing means that somewhere the individual's name will be in the chart, and the results will be available to a limited number of other people. Anonymous testing means that there is a coded identifier without reference to a name. This is really important for many people because it removes the fear of others finding out a positive result and possibly misusing that information by discriminatory acts against the infected individual.

Will the Result Be Reported to the State Public Health Department?

Some states require reporting for an HIV+ status and AIDS, others only for AIDS. *HIV+* means that the client is without symptoms but is infectious. *AIDS* means that there are signs, symptoms, or infections as specified by the Center for Disease Control (CDC) or that the CD4 or T4 cell count has dropped below 200.

What Support Systems Are Available?

This is a crucial question. Clients may be terrified of telling anyone about the results for a number of reasons. There may be fear that they have infected someone else, knowledge of family negative feelings toward HIV, and dread that they may be isolated and abandoned.

Telling their family or life partner may change their lives inexorably. It is a step that must be taken as thoughtfully and carefully as possible. They may wish, and should be encouraged to seek, outside support from the beginning through a local HIV support group, but do remember that at some time their nearest and dearest will need to know. From the beginning, protective measures must be taken to prevent further transmission and spread to their loved ones.

Where Are the Local Community Resources?

The health professional should have a basic knowledge of the available resources before recommending them. What is good for one may not be for another.

A young pregnant woman may not feel comfortable in a largely gay male organization, and the feelings would probably be the same in reverse. Do propose community resources appropriate to the needs of the client. Provide addresses, telephone numbers, and the particular services that the organizations offer.

Will the Test Hurt?

No.

What Is Done?

Blood is drawn from the arm and is subjected to an enzyme-linked immunosorbent assay (ELISA) test. It detects the antibodies caused by HIV. If the test detects the antibodies, a second ELISA will be performed. If that is also positive, a confirmatory test called the Western Blot will then be done. Today both these tests have a 99.9% accuracy rate. Some false positive results do occur and may happen when chronic hepatitis, alcohol-related liver disease, or collagen vascular disease are present.

When Should I Be Tested?

Any time. However, do remember that there is a window period following actual transmission when the ELISA test cannot detect the antibodies. The majority of people will have detectable antibodies within 3 months after transmission and almost all of the remainder will have them within 6 months. It is vitally important to remind people that although the antibodies are not detectable in these first months, the person is infectious and can transmit the virus.

If I Am HIV+, How Will the Law Protect Me?

It is imperative that the counselor know all the HIV/AIDS state laws. A handout with a summary of state laws and community, state, and national resource telephone hotline numbers is very helpful.

Will There Be Financial Help for Me?

Yes, clients can receive financial help through health insurance, Medicare, Medicaid, Social Security Disability Insurance, Supplemental Security Income, and Ryan White monies.

Why Am I Doing This?

Early diagnosis means early assessment; access to clinical trials; improved medical management, which often means a longer life span; an improved sense of personal control by living a healthier life style; and preventing the infection of someone else.

How Long Before I Receive the Results?

This varies according to where the test is done. It can be anywhere from 5 to 10 days in public health clinics and 2 to 5 days through a private physician's office.

What Happens When I Am Tested?

Clients will meet with a counselor privately. The conversation is always confidential. The counselor will ask a number of questions about past and present sexual history, sexual practices and other at-risk behaviors, how much clients know about HIV/AIDS, and what a positive result would mean to them. Also, if the clients are HIV+, they will be asked if they would be willing to identify those people with whom they have had sexual or injecting-drug-sharing relationships so that those persons can be informed that they may also be at risk for HIV and should be tested. The counselor will explain the purpose and reliability of the tests, provide clients with information regarding HIV, discuss safer behaviors, ask clients to read and sign an informed consent form, and ask clients to make an appointment to return to receive the results. Clients should also be given a telephone number and contact person to call for further information and support during the waiting period.

What Is Informed Consent?

A written or oral informed consent asks the client's permission to perform the procedure. It must be obtained in many states from the person to be tested or from the guardian of a minor. The form is different in each state and should be read carefully and not signed until every part of it is understood and accepted. When your clients' questions are answered to their satisfaction, they may then choose to be tested. Then comes the waiting period. However short or long, this time, similar to waiting for any other diagnoses that may be life limiting, is when clients need understanding, sensitivity, and support.

WAITING FOR THE RESULTS

For many people, this is a time of indescribable anxiety, and it often produces a veritable roller coaster of emotions from anger to regret to depression. Indeed, suicides have occurred during this period, which seems a tragic waste. Our role, to quote a beautiful, practical hospice nun, is "to be there, to be sensitive, and to be silent." Allow the ventilation of feelings, discourage physical bodily harm, and provide nonjudgmental support. Encourage exercise, food, liquids, and rest. Discourage increased alcohol or drug intake. Most of all, walk this path beside them, validate their feelings, acknowledge their fears, and remind them that if they are HIV+, this is not by any means a death sentence. It is remarkable that many people do not return to receive their test results. Counselors must encourage their clients to do this, otherwise the clients' health status will remain unknown, their risky behaviors may continue, and other lives may be put at risk.

THE RESULTS: HIV+

Counseling should be done in person and never over the telephone. It is always confidential. If the results are positive, clients will need time to adjust to this. It is important that the HIV pre- and posttest counselor should make at least one follow-up appointment, and more if necessary. The reason for this is that clients frequently fall into a period of "tunnel hearing" that generally lasts about 48 hours. Tunnel hearing hears only the positive result, not the positive outcomes. Feelings of loss are high and are often expressed through anger, anxiety, rage, betrayal, denial, shock, and behavior threatening to self and to others.

I well remember a newly diagnosed young man who rushed into my office holding a gun to his temple, screaming "I'm positive, it's all over, and I'm killing myself now!" Having someone shoot himself in my office was definitely not on that day's agenda! I took some deep breaths, mentally counting down from 100, and was eternally grateful that my voice did not squeak when I spoke and asked him if he would like to sit down and tell me what had happened. He visibly calmed, sat down, and started talking. By enormous good fortune, one of our volunteer physicians who specializes in HIV was in the building and was able to gently ease in, remove the gun, and provide expert available treatment options for a man who is alive and healthy today and who has become a devoted volunteer, educator, and friend.

Being allowed to ventilate in a safe place is the beginning of the person taking control of the disease rather than the disease taking control of the person. Physical manifestations of loss will also occur and include heightened blood pressure and heartbeat, decreased ability to concentrate, tightening of the throat, nausea, tears, sighing, sweating palms, possible retching and vomiting, diarrhea, and a loss of equilibrium (Lamerton, 1973).

Unfortunately, the counselor may only have one opportunity to give the results and to provide posttest counseling. This is never an ideal situation, so it is really important to make the most of it. As mentioned earlier in the chapter, individuals frequently do not return for their HIV+ tests results, and those who do may not fully understand the information that is being given to them. As much time as possible should be spent with the client, and feedback should be elicited frequently. Posttest counseling should include

- giving the results in a tranquil, private location, calmly and supportively.
- assessing and addressing the client's knowledge regarding HIV/AIDS.
- the provision of clearly written, informative materials.
- a resource list of local infectious disease physicians working in the HIV/AIDS arena and suggesting an early appointment with the physician so that blood screening and a physical examination can be done.
- explaining the improved life expectancy if medical intervention occurs early. Remember, the explanation must be geared to the client's language and comprehension level—illustrations are often as helpful as words.
- detailed information regarding "safer" behaviors, particularly demonstrating how to use condoms, both male and female, and, if appropriate, how to clean drug apparatus.

- reminding women that there is the possibility that their babies may become infected if they are pregnant or choose to become pregnant. They should also be informed of the very good outcome for babies if mothers receive AZT during pregnancy. They should be advised of where they should seek treatment.
- a suggestion that family planning be used, using local family planning clinics.
- an explanation regarding, and encouragement to use, substance abuse rehabilitative programs.
- reminders that nutrition, exercise, rest, and healthy lifestyles are the first steps in taking personal responsibility and control.
- a reminder that AIDS must be reported by state health departments to the CDC. However, each state has different requirements regarding the reporting of HIV, so counselors should know the law of their individual state.
- a request that clients notify all past sexual contacts or injecting-drug-using people with whom they have shared needles. This may be physically and emotionally impossible for clients. If it is, the local health department is able to do so. In some states, contact tracing or partner notification is mandatory.
- an outline of available clinical trials and a resource list with national, state, and local HIV/AIDS hotlines.
- a comprehensive list of community resources and list of the times and places of available support groups.
- a list of HIV/AIDS psychotherapeutic counselors for individual therapy.

HIV-NEGATIVE TESTS

It is important that posttest counseling also occur for those who test negative. Clients may be genuinely negative or the test may have happened during the window period, or the test may be indeterminate. Posttest HIV negative counseling should include

- a review of the test results.
- a determination as to whether the client was recently at risk for HIV exposure and, if so, a reminder that being tested in 6 months time is the recommended course of action. If the tests are still negative at that time and no further possible HIV exposure has occurred, the client should be presumed to be negative.
- if there is a further waiting period, no donation of blood or plasma until those test results are received.
- a review of risk behaviors, safer behaviors, and, if available, a resource group for the "worried well."
- a strong reminder that although they are negative, this does not mean that future risky behaviors will continue to have the same result.

DISCLOSURE

After the decision to be tested, the decision as to whom to tell causes inactions and actions that can cause regret, disillusionment, and harm for the rest of a person's life. Inappropriate disclosure has caused the loss of jobs, insurance, health insurance, family, friends, life partners, and ultimately of basic survival needs. It has caused individuals to self-isolate and self-abandon themselves. When the mind is in turmoil, sometimes the mouth goes into high gear. Discourage this!

Questions clients should ask themselves are the following:

- What is the attitude and knowledge regarding HIV/AIDS of your immediate family, life partner, spouse, friend, physician, and clergyperson?
- Who of the above are nonjudgmental, discreet, and supportive?
- What are the formal and informal policies and beliefs regarding HIV/AIDS where you work?
- Does your health insurance policy disclaim preexisting conditions?
- Do you know the attitudes of the owner, tenants, and neighbors toward HIV/AIDS where you rent or own your home?
- Does your state have antidiscriminatory HIV/AIDS laws and are they implemented?
- Does your culture and ethnic background support PWAs, or is there denial and reprehension?
- Are you able to ask for help or are you always the supporter or the linchpin of the family?

Disclosure can have some disconcerting and long-term ramifications and should be undertaken thoughtfully and carefully.

Several years ago a couple in their mid-70s came for counseling. The wife had received blood transfusions during open-heart surgery in Miami in 1983. By 1987, she was exhibiting continuing symptoms of low-grade fever, tremendous fatigue, and some weight loss. She had seen several gerontologists who had examined her and sent her for a barrage of tests but never thought to test her for HIV antibodies. She was, after all, from their perception, the wrong age and in the right relationship. She eventually saw an infectious disease physician in 1989 who discovered her HIV+ status and also found that her husband was infected. This was devastating enough, but an ongoing saga of events was to follow. They lived in a well-known retirement village and were terrified that the residents would find out and condemn and isolate them. They asked their three adult children who lived out of state to come and visit them. At a family gathering, the parents told their children about their infection. The eldest daughter was furious and screamed at her parents for "deceiving" her and putting their grandchildren at risk. She angrily told them they would never see their grandchildren again and pulled her husband out of the apartment, and true to her word that was the last they were to see of her. The remaining son and daughter, both married and without children, were wonderfully supportive but had jobs that prevented them from visiting frequently. When the wife became very ill, she joined a hospice program and begged that the large and very identifiable waste disposal van not come into the retirement village to collect her waste disposal container as she was fearful of the other residents' reactions and afraid that they could be forced out their condominium. She died comfortably but depressed, afraid for her husband and sorrowing over the loss of her daughter and grandchildren. Should she have told the family? Yes; but it may have helped to have had a counselor present who could have tried to educate their daughter, who was obviously ignorant regarding HIV. Sadly, everyone lost.

Another couple in their mid-50s, both health care professionals, outgoing, vital, and isolated, also came for counseling. They had lived in a rural area of a southern state where everyone knows everyone and is often related to one another. When his HIV+ status was discovered, they sold everything, bought a sailboat, and moved to Florida—the American Dream! They told their secret to no one and kept in touch with family and friends only by telephone. They neither visited home nor invited anyone to visit them. By the time they sought counseling, his elderly mother was becoming increasingly suspicious that something was wrong with her beloved son, and she wanted to see him now. They spent an hour identifying friends and relatives who might be supportive, and, by role-playing, came up with three with whom they felt a high level of trust. Worst-case scenarios were discussed if these individuals proved not to be supportive and it was decided that there seemed to be more to gain than to lose by telling them. We talked about the method of the telling, that is, by phone, visiting, or inviting these people down individually. They decided on the latter so that they would have the reassurance and safety of their own surroundings. The first and subsequent visits were wonderfully successful. Eventually, he told his mother and two adult daughters from a previous marriage. The most incredible support continued until his peaceful death in his own home surrounded by people who loved him.

Disclosure may occur later rather than sooner, according to the individual's own attitudes and those of his or her emotional and medical support systems. The results of disclosure are unpredictable and are molded by many factors. It is always risky, but the risks can have extraordinarily good outcomes.

One of the most important people in the medical support system is the physician. The right physician is the key to developing and maintaining the best physical health and emotional well-being. Not all physicians are willing to work with PWAs, or, when they are, are not always knowledgeable regarding HIV disease, HIV medications, or advances in HIV research. Choosing the right physician will make a difference in the quality and quantity of the care provided, will increase the opportunity to receive up-to-date treatment options, and should produce a cooperative partnership of care between the client and the doctor. Options are more limited when care is provided by primary health care clinics, health maintenance organizations, or preferred provider organizations rather than private health insurance.

Organizations such as the American Medical Association and Burrowes Wellcome (1992) and the journal *Positively Aware* (Chavez, 1993) have written excellent guidelines for choosing a physician, some of which are reflected in the following suggestions for your clients.

CHOOSING A PHYSICIAN

The client should

- ask for recommendations for a physician who is an expert in HIV/AIDS care and treatment. Ask friends, family physician or dentist, or the local medical

association or call the national AIDS hotline for a list of physicians in their area (English, 1-800-342-AIDS; Spanish, 1-800-344-7432).
• contact an infectious disease physician or immunologist if there is no expert on HIV in their area.
• find out their fee structure, if they accept insurance, if they accept Medicaid, if they have a sliding scale fee structure, and what their payment terms are.
• find out if they are knowledgeable regarding clinical trials and if they are part of a community research initiative.
• look for accessible location, transportation, and office hours.
• find out if they are accepting new patients at this time.
• ask for an initial interview and make an appointment.

The initial interview is important. It is the first step in establishing trust and should be the beginning of a long and harmonious relationship. Each client deserves the very best that medicine has to offer. To ensure that clients receive it, here are some suggestions for the interview.

THE INTERVIEW

Before the interview, clients should write down all the questions that they want to ask, thus ensuring that nothing is forgotten. They should take with them any current medical records, including recent results of x-rays, scans, mammograms, and pap smears. Clients should take along a friend to boost their morale and to take notes. They should observe the staff and waiting room. Is the staff pleasant and welcoming? Is the waiting room clean and bright? Do they have to wait long? When they meet the physician, they should feel a sense of mutual respect and feel comfortable that this will be a long-term partnership. The first interview is usually lengthy because of history taking, a physical examination, and probably blood tests. Do they have time to ask and receive answers to their questions, or do they feel rushed? Can they comfortably discuss any issues, whether they address sexual preference, drug use, relationships aside from that with their spouse or life or sexual partner, present or future pregnancies, or STDs? Do they feel confident that they will receive the most current medical treatment and that they will be offered choices and options? Does the physician use language that they can understand? They should ask which HIV monitoring schedule the physician follows and when the next appointment will be and write it down.

The art of living with HIV includes taking charge, becoming an educated consumer, trusting one's physician, monitoring and evaluating one's choices, being aware of all the available resources locally and nationally, and using clinical trials if one is eligible and willing to do so.

CLINICAL TRIALS

The role of clinical trials cannot be overstated. The search for a safe and effective vaccine is an international health priority according to the National Institute of Allergy and Infectious Diseases, the Food and Drug Administration, the CDC, and other federal agencies. Quoting from the AIDS Clinical Trials Information Service brochure (1993), "AIDS clinical trials evaluate experimental drugs and other therapies for adults and children at all stages of HIV infection—from patients who are HIV positive with no symptoms to those with various symptoms of AIDS."

A growing array of trials are now available and can be found throughout the country in teaching and community hospitals and physicians who belong to community-based initiatives. The decision to participate in trials should be approached thoughtfully. Questions clients should ask are "Why should I take the medication(s)?" "What are the side effects?" "What will it do?" "Will I have to travel far, and when should I start?"

There is no known cure for HIV/AIDS yet, and the decision to take any medications is not an easy one to make. At least 5% of the HIV population worldwide is living longer and healthier without any medical intervention other than regular checkups. Why they are living well is under intensive research, and there are no clear-cut answers at present. What is known is that antiretrovirals (drugs that fight the retrovirus) have made a significant difference to the thousands of people who have taken them by boosting their immune system and improving their health. The first useful antiretroviral was a drug called Retrovir or zidovudine (still better known as AZT). Originally it was used on its own; now it is often used in combination with a number of different medications. The combination therapies (using two or more drugs) may be more effective than using a single drug.

As can be seen by the material already covered in this chapter, being HIV+ brings forth a complexity of needs that affect the physical, emotional, psychosocial, and spiritual health of infected individuals and their loved ones. From a clinical point of view, it is essential that the health care professional understands what an HIV+ result represents.

WHAT DOES IT MEAN TO BE HIV+?

When HIV enters the body, it attacks the immune system by invading what are called CD4 cells, more commonly referred to as T4 cells. Infected cells then replicate within the T4 cell until the cell erupts, releasing the infected cells to attack other T4 cells. HIV attacks other cells of the immune system as well, but the T4 cells are the body's "fighter" cells that fight off diseases and infections, and as their numbers diminish, the immune system becomes weaker. It is at this stage that HIV usually leads into AIDS. If there is early intervention, good medical treatment, and the development of a healthy lifestyle, individuals should live longer and better, with the possibility of a cure being discovered in their lifetimes.

In a healthy adult, HIV disease manifests itself in four stages that occur over a period of many years. Different institutions and individuals use different methods to define the stages of HIV progression. Here are excerpts from two of them.

The CDC (1986) defined the stages as the following: Group I—acute infection, a mononucleosis-like illness associated with seroconversion for HIV antibody; Group II—asymptomatic infection, an absence of signs or symptoms of HIV infection;

Group III—persistent generalized lymphodenopathy, lymph node enlargements of more than 1 centimeter at two or more extrainguinal sites persisting for more than 3 months; and Group IV—other diseases: Subgroup A—constitutional disease, one or more episodes of fever persisting for more than 1 month, involuntary weight loss below 10%, and diarrhea persisting for more than 1 month; Subgroup B—neurologic disease, one or more of dementia, myelopathy, or peripheral neuropathy; Subgroup C—secondary infectious diseases, the diagnosis of an infectious disease associated with HIV.

An article in the January/February 1993 issue of *HIVFRONTLINE* (McKusick, 1993) suggested that the stages are the following: (a) asymptomatic, (b) single-symptom or single opportunistic infection, (c) multiple, overlapping, and recurrent symptoms, and (d) end stage. To make the labels less clinical and more "person with HIV"–centered, the article suggested changing them to (a) no illness, (b) discrete illness, (c) cascade of illness, and (d) end of life.

One has to be extraordinarily careful with any kind of staging and labeling as each individual is unique and rarely follows established paths. The stages should be used as signposts, not as tablets of stone!

Now is a good time to examine the process and challenge of the disease and develop step-by-step interventions.

Asymptomatic or No Illness

After the first shock and depression have worn off, equilibrium has been restored, and a medical monitoring and treatment plan has been established, life should return to some normalcy.

Counselors can

- help develop support systems and find support groups that are knowledgeable and upbeat. Although it is rare, some groups and facilitators have agendas that are not constructive but are self-serving and manipulative.
- provide nonjudgmental listening.
- encourage safer behaviors. Even if a sexual partner is infected, unprotected sex may cause a crossing of HIV strains or the transmission of other diseases.
- recognize that feelings, reactions, and responses are a roller coaster ride of ups and downs. They can change from hour to hour and day to day.
- remember that other life events are occurring simultaneously—divorces, separations, job losses, illness of children, deaths of friends and family. None of them stop because of HIV, and all will need intervention.
- understand the coping style of the individual and provide strategies that match that style. The normally organized person copes very differently than the normally disorganized person, and the "internalizer" is different from the "externalizer"—there is no "one true way"!
- address fears as they arise. If you do not know the answer to a question, don't be afraid to say so, but do say that you will try to find the answer.
- inspire motivation by assisting the development of short- and medium-range goals that can be as simple as a walk on the beach or as complex as planning an African photographic safari; as necessary as writing a will or as rewarding

as seeing friends and family for whom there was never enough time. Ask your clients; they will know what they want and need to do.

- encourage the use of technical, social, spiritual, and caring skills to help others. Thousands of PWAs worldwide have found that being infected has inspired them to undertake tasks that they never would have believed possible.
- discourage a "victim" mentality. Frequently, people who are labeled adapt to the label. *Victim* is a negative, downbeat word.
- teach the gifts of guided imagery, visualization, affirmation, relaxation exercises, and deep-breathing stress reducers.
- suggest massage therapy.
- investigate state and local resources for financial support, transportation, housing, and food banks.
- support a healthy lifestyle that includes exercise, a nutritious diet, and plenty of rest.
- use humor in any way possible—jokes, cartoons, videos, movies, television comedies, books—anything that appeals. The power of laughter should never be underestimated.

Understand that you, the counselor, may become frustrated and that positive solutions are not always possible. Be vigorous in suggesting medical assessment for every sign and symptom.

Single-Symptom or Single Opportunistic Infection—Discrete Illness

After the initial infection, years may pass before there is a sign, symptom, or opportunistic infection. During this time, clients usually move from a time of chaos into a time of picking up their lives and moving forward. The disease is relegated to the back burner, and a certain amount of healthy denial exists. The fact of an HIV+ status has very little emotional power and becomes somewhat of an intellectual icon: It exists, it's not hurting me, so what's the problem?

The problem comes when the very first sign, symptom, or opportunistic infection occurs, and the T4 cell count becomes unstable. There is a rapid confrontation with reality, and a secondary phenomenon of anticipatory grief occurs. There is an almost immediate and often overwhelming feeling of inevitability manifested in fear, anxiety, depression, anger, panic, and social withdrawal. There is a searching and yearning for the wellness that existed such a short time before.

The health care system, family, friends, counselors, and God may be blamed for what is perceived as a failure of self and the system. The individual's self-esteem plummets, which may be accompanied by lassitude and indifference to life itself. Counselors can:

- encourage the expression of feelings by nonadvisory, nonjudgmental listening.
- explore the feelings and provide honest feedback.
- recognize that the client may be a multiple mourner who has seen family and friends die from AIDS and now sees him- or herself on a death spiral. This is almost always very scary.
- teach stress management tactics, which are detailed in chapter 10.

- assist in reevaluating life goals. Dividing them into separate lists of needs and wants often provides an accessible visual and emotional pathway to prioritize and accomplish them.
- suggest the completion of any unfinished business, whatever it is.
- help assess present and future financial needs and the availability of assistance within the community.
- discourage the overuse of alcohol and nicotine.
- assist in reviewing legal needs such as the appointment of a health care surrogate, personal power of attorney, living wills, and wills.
- evaluate the probable health care needs now and in the future pertaining to housing, caretaking, case management, and continuing medical treatment.
- encourage compliance with medication regimens.
- research other treatment options.
- support the surrounding family—everyone will feel something.

During this stage, hospitalization may be necessary. If it is, there are some things that can be done to make the stay less overwhelming and more empowering.

Hospitalization

Before leaving home. Clients should stop the newspaper delivery, arrange with a friend to care for their house and car, and let neighbors know that someone will be coming in and out. They should store valuable items such as jewelry, credit cards, insurance documents, and so forth, and let a family member know where they are. Child care should be arranged. Clients should leave written directions regarding favorite foods, stories, and outings, and the telephone numbers and addresses of the pediatrician and relatives, as well as written instructions for pet and plant care. A key should be left with a trusted neighbor in the event of an emergency. Current bills should be paid, or the client should arrange for someone to do this for them. The client should pack a suitcase. For almost everyone, going to the hospital is a time of concern and anxiety. Taking familiar things helps to restore a sense of order and comfort. Packing the suitcase is therefore important!

Packing the suitcase. The client should take tried, true, and comfortable nightclothes and footwear; definitely a teddy bear or equivalent; familiar soap, perfume, aftershave, body lotion, deodorant, toothbrush, toothpaste, and lip balm; cash in small denominations for newspapers, magazines, candies, and television; portable radio and cassette player; favorite music, relaxation tapes, and cassette books; something small and familiar such as a photograph, pillow, or book; address book; diary or journal to keep track of events; cheap ballpoint pens; wristwatch or small travel clock; hard candy; the book they always wanted to read but never had the time to; health insurance and legal documents; and a writing pad, to write all those letters that have piled up and to keep a note of all the questions that need answers.

With good treatment intervention, the reduction of stress, and effective support systems, the individual usually bounces back from this episode and is ready to live the good life once again. Indeed, there may be several of these episodes followed by a return to relatively good health and comfortable living. At some time, the signs, symptoms, and opportunistic infections almost certainly will increase; however, this is so different with each person that attempting to name a time frame is impossible.

Multiple, Overlapping, and Recurrent Symptoms—Cascade of Illness

This stage usually presents a diversity of symptoms and concurrent infections. It often means an intensifying of aggressive therapies, less effective medications, a physical world that is growing smaller because of decreasing mobility, and an increasing dependence on medical technology, health staff, and support systems. Independence is one of the West's most treasured belief systems, founded on Judeo-Christian values and a culture that correlates who one is with what one does. Dependence on others is extraordinarily difficult for anyone, but this is particularly so when most of those affected are young, often vital contributors to society who are used to developing their own choices and options. This is a time when the health team and the individual's needs may be perceived differently. The team may aggressively increase medical intervention, whereas the individual may wish to review his or her current and future needs and seek different solutions. The counselor can:

- recognize that this is a time of mood swings coupled with extreme fatigue.
- organize social activities at a time when the fatigue factor is not as severe. Clients know which parts of the day are better than others.
- listen to the client's needs and attempt to resolve them. This often means negotiation and advocacy between the medical team, family, or friends.
- anticipate that the client may express an intention to commit suicide. By asking open-ended questions, it is usually possible to find out the underlying fears. Often people are not afraid of death but are afraid of the dying process and of severe pain. Talking about dying and pain management can cause a huge reduction of fear.
- suggest asking the physician for a low dose of psychotropic medication, which will reduce irritability and depression and improve rest and well-being.
- encourage friends to provide practical support such as cooking meals, providing transportation, cleaning the house or apartment, tidying the garden or yard, reading the newspaper, writing letters, and doing the laundry, walking the dog, or taking a child to the playground.
- if no caretaker is available, organize a visitation roster of family or friends and provide some basic education for infection management, transfers from the bed to the wheelchair or commode, and bathing and feeding.
- try to help resolve family disputes when there is estrangement. Families who are able to resolve their differences and participate in the care of a loved one are infinitely rewarded compared with those who remain estranged.
- as death approaches, find out where the client would prefer to die. Some people feel much safer in hospital surrounded by high tech. Others would prefer to be in the safety and comfort of their own home. If the choice is to stay at home or in a less cure-motivated environment, a hospice program may be the answer.

HOSPICES

Hospices emphasize the quality of living until the moment of death. To do this, hospice programs believe in efficient, loving care that provides comprehensive pain and symptom management and emotional, spiritual, and social support to terminally ill persons and their families.

Hospices have no age limit and are available through Medicare, Medicaid, and private insurance plans. Most patient care is delivered in the home by an interdisciplinary team composed of physicians, nurses, home health assistants, pastoral counselors, social workers, and occupational speech, nutrition, and physical therapists. Many hospice programs have units within nursing homes or acute care hospitals or are free-standing. All of them are furnished to be as homelike as possible and have 24-hour visiting hours that often include pets. Trained volunteers are a wonderful part of hospices and provide compassionate support for everyone. Hospices will provide care around the clock in the home if that is either a patient or a family need.

Hospices are not sad places, but cheerful, honest, and compassionate. They provide intensive care delivered in a different way.

CONCLUSION

This chapter has presented a generic overview of some of the issues that arise with HIV/AIDS. It has shown a progression of the disease and some of the needs that occur at various stages of the disease.

HIV/AIDS is a complex disease that must be seen within the larger context of the individual, family, support systems, community, nation, and the world. The social issues that surround HIV/AIDS are a continuum of other social issues that have to be addressed locally, nationally, and globally if we really wish to have a healthy people. Crime, poverty, STDs, substance abuse, neglect, abuse, prejudice, high school dropouts, teenage pregnancies, incest, rape, and indifference are but a few of the challenges that confront us. HIV forces us to look at ingrained societal tragedies that will change only if each of us recognizes that we can make a difference if we choose to make a difference. The next chapter will address the special needs of women and children who are extraordinarily affected by the HIV/AIDS pandemic.

REFERENCES

American Medical Association. *Choosing your physician* [Brochure].

Bach, R. (1970). *Jonathan Livingston Seagull.* New York: Avon Books.

Centers for Disease Control. (1986). *Current trends: Classification system for human T-lymphotropic virus type III/lymphadenopathy associated virus infections.* Washington, DC: Community Health Network.

Centers for Disease Control and Prevention, Health Resources and Service Administration, National Institutes of Health. (1993). *Surgeon General's report to the*

American public on HIV infection and AIDS (1993-534-369). Washington, DC: U.S. Government Printing Office.

Chavez, C. (1993). Starting off on the right foot: How to choose a physician. *Positively Aware, Spring,* 5.

Grossman, R. (1992). *How to work with your doctor to fight HIV* [Brochure]. Burroughs Wellcome.

Health & Rehabilitative Services. (1990). *About living with HIV* [Brochure].

Hinton, J. (1972). *Dying* (2nd ed.). Middlesex, England: Penguin Books.

Lamerton, R. (1973). *Care of the dying.* East Sussex, England: Garden City Press.

McKusick, L. (Ed.). (1993). Riding the HIV roller coaster: Counselling and care in later-stage illness. *HIVFRONTLINE, 11,* 4.

National Institute of Allergy and Infectious Disease. (1994). *AIDS vaccine.* Washington, DC: U.S. Government Printing Office.

U.S. Department of Health and Human Services. (1993). *AIDS Clinical Trials Information Service* [Brochure]. Washington, DC: Author.

3

Women and Children:
The Traditionally Underserved

Evidence suggests that by the time a woman is diagnosed with AIDS she'll die four to six times faster than a man. All too often, a woman isn't diagnosed until she gets pregnant, her baby is born HIV infected or she is hospitalized with an opportunistic disease associated with the onset of AIDS.

—Fleur Sack, *A Romance to Die For*

Throughout the world, young women of childbearing age are the fastest growing group becoming infected with HIV. Since January 1992, close to one half of the new AIDS cases worldwide have been diagnosed in women. It is estimated that in 1995 there were 3 million women and 500,000 children infected with HIV. In the next half decade, 10–15 million women will become infected (Grubman & Oleske, 1993). HIV/AIDS has become a family disease that affects the community and society as a whole.

In the United States, women mirror the rest of the world and are also the fastest growing HIV-infected group. In New York City, the opportunistic infections associated with AIDS are now the leading killers of women between the ages of 25 and 34. Because of the long latency period between HIV infection and the onset of symptoms, most young women were likely infected with HIV as adolescents. Although the annual incidence of AIDS among children and women of childbearing age in the United States has been increasing for most racial and ethnic groups, it has been persistently higher among women of color and Hispanics than any other group (Hicks & Hirsch, 1990).

Many of those who are infected with HIV are from socially and economically disadvantaged groups who may already suffer from feelings of alienation and low self-esteem. HIV/AIDS may just be one more bad thing that happens to them. Their needs reach well beyond health care and HIV management and may also include substance abuse treatment, housing, child care, transportation, and respite services, to name but a few.

Many families affected by, or at risk for, HIV have a history of drug dependence or involvement with drug users and require drug treatment intervention and ongoing sobriety support to remove the drug-based link to HIV/AIDS. HIV-affected families require comprehensive health and social services designed to maintain the family unit while providing access to health care (National Community AIDS Partnership, 1992).

Recognizing and understanding the multiple and diverse issues that confront women, adolescents, and children infected and affected by HIV is the only way to ensure that comprehensive intervention, diagnosis, and treatment are provided in a timely, positive, compassionate, and efficient manner.

WOMEN AND HIV: THE CHALLENGE

Women around the world, infected or affected, often share similar challenges regardless of their age, language, culture, and ethnicity. The challenges are so numerous that it is impossible to identify them all. The health care professional will find that the list includes, but is not limited to, the following: exclusion from or limited access to medical research programs; limited access to health care systems; difficulty in proving eligibility for disability; access to family planning programs; that do not include HIV education, unsafe sexual practices, protective nontoxic barrier methods; and insufficient or inappropriate drug rehabilitation programs.

It does not stop there. There is a need for education and age-based care and treatment for older infected women, women-specific support groups, foster and adoptive parents for children, child care centers that are not afraid to knowingly look after HIV-infected kids, and health care professionals who work with and advocate for dying children. Let us begin the journey with research programs designed for women.

MEDICAL RESEARCH PROGRAMS

As late as 1990, women in the United States and the rest of the world had little involvement with HIV research studies, which were offered to and performed on White men (Diaz, 1991). This was not just a problem of HIV/AIDS-related research. Many clinical trials on drugs have excluded women from the research protocols, regardless of the disease, and in many cases recommendations for drug use are based on their safety, efficiency, and efficacy in White men.

In addition to the lack of access to research protocols, there is a problem in attracting members of racial and ethnic minorities to participate. Distrust of the system by and feelings of uneasiness in members of racial and ethnic minorities at being involved in research are often cited as the reasons for not participating.

Nevertheless, progress is being made, albeit slowly and haltingly. Recent and exciting results have come from a study conducted by the Pediatric AIDS Clinical Trials Group of the National Institute of Allergy and Infectious Diseases (NIAID) in collaboration with the National de la Santé et de la Récherches Medicale and Agencé National de Récherches sur le SIDA in France (J. Lange, 1994). Use of the drug zidovudine, more commonly known as AZT, was initiated with pregnant women between 14 and 34 weeks gestation and continued to the end of their pregnancy. There was a substantial decrease in the transmission rate of HIV to their babies. This is excellent news. As trials for women are becoming more available, it is really important to access these trials early.

Before anyone participates in a clinical trials program, they should have as much knowledge as possible regarding the objective of the trials, the possible side effects, any associated expenses, and what will be required of them.

Clinical trials are not for everyone. Regular appointments must be kept, blood and urine samples are usually taken at each visit, there may be uncomfortable side effects, and the prescribed medications must be taken at a specific time in a specific way. People in research programs should receive a lot of support and encouragement from friends and health professionals. The benefits cannot be overstressed. Not only may there be improved short- and long-term good health for the individual, but the knowledge gained will help many others. Eventually, research will surely find a vaccine to prevent HIV and a medication for its cure. Without research, neither of these hoped-for events can happen.

ACCESS TO HEALTH CARE SYSTEMS

Access is the name of the game for early diagnosis and treatment. Lack of access occurs for a variety of reasons. For instance, there may be a limited knowledge of HIV or the belief that it cannot "happen to me" or "that's someone else's problem, not mine," causing signs and symptoms to be ignored and to remain undiagnosed; the fear of family and friends finding out the diagnosis, with the possibility of subsequent stigma resulting in isolation and abandonment; a large family of young children where Mom, the traditional core of the family, has her hands full looking after them and little time or energy to take care of herself; HIV/AIDS clinics at a distance and transportation difficult or unavailable; children's day care financially impossible, deterring women from seeking treatment; lack of drug treatment programs directed toward HIV-infected women; limited or no health insurance; long waits in public health clinics and inconvenient appointment hours; sometimes insensitive treatment that results in an understandable refusal to return; cultural attitudes toward HIV; fear of the loss of control of one's life; and fear of the loss of one's children and the ultimate loss of social support systems (Perez, 1991).

CONQUERING THE ACCESS CHALLENGE

For anything to work, it must have the participation, support, and trust of the people who are directly involved—the infected and the affected. All too often, health care professionals believe they know the best course of action for others without recognizing that a woman's health needs may be the last thing on her agenda. Treatment and care agendas have to match to be effective.

Some of the things that help are the development of representative community groups to plan present and future needs; the building of comprehensive community-based women's health care centers that provide an array of services, including culturally sensitive and nonsexist HIV education and services; pre- and posttest HIV counseling; HIV testing; HIV treatment and care; family planning; mental health counseling; choices in pregnancy; pregnancy counseling; counseling and treatment for sexually transmitted diseases (STDs); tuberculosis screening and treatment; child care; drug rehabilitation; and legal aid and transportation all available under one roof. Transportation can make or break such a program. A young mother, holding her sickly, coughing, and crying 18-month-old baby, shrieked at health care providers, "You all keep on telling me what to do and where I can get help, but none of you tell me how to get there!" Transportation may be the most important factor in accessing care, and both volunteers and money may be needed to provide it.

HIV/AIDS is a costly illness. It is gradually becoming a well-managed disease of prolonged wellness when diagnosis and treatment occur early in its infection. However, there will usually come a time when extra financial support is needed, and one way to obtain this is through Social Security.

UNDERSTANDING SOCIAL SECURITY REGULATIONS

The good news is that Social Security regulations have changed (U.S. Department of Health and Human Services, 1993), making it easier to qualify for Supplemental Security Income (SSI) and to receive Social Security Disability Insurance (SSDI). (SSI and SSDI are also described in chapter 5.) In the past, to qualify for SSI, applicants had to pass a "functional limitations" test to prove their disability. The test was usually very confusing to the applicant.

Under the old regulations, persons with HIV qualified for benefits if they had one or more illnesses that were on the Social Security Administration's list of illnesses considered disabling. These illnesses are called "stand-alone" illnesses. For instance, *Pneumocystis carinii* pneumonia (PCP) was considered a stand-alone illness. If applicants could prove that they had PCP, they would probably be identified as being disabled and would then receive benefits (Cohn, 1993).

The regulations, which originally listed 32 stand-alone illnesses, now list 41. The bad news is that if "an applicant does not meet the exact description of the illness, they will not qualify under the 'stand alone' guidelines, but instead will have to meet the new Functional Limitation test" (Cohn, 1993, p. 6). However, the new test is simpler and more generous to the applicant and will be applied to cases that are already pending.

Women-specific stand-alone illnesses are the following:

- carcinoma of the cervix that has spread to surrounding tissues
- condyloma or genital warts that are ulcerated or quite large and not responding to treatment
- genital herpes lasting 1 month or longer
- pelvic inflammatory disease (PID) that has required hospitalization or intravenous antibiotic treatment three or more times a year. PID occurs when a sexually transmitted bacteria such as gonorrhea or chlamydia causes an infection in the uterus, the ovaries, or both.
- vulvovaginal candidiasis, better known as a vaginal yeast infection, that has

ulcerated and does not respond to vaginal creams and suppositories such as Monistat or antifungal medications such as Ketoconazale

QUALIFYING FOR DISABILITY

The illnesses may not be severe enough to meet the stand-alone guidelines, but do not let the client be disheartened. There are other qualifications that, if met, can prove that HIV infection is chronic and functionally limiting (words to keep on remembering!) If need can be proved, benefits should be forthcoming.

Chronic Illness Needs

A chronic illness means that an illness has lasted at least 2 weeks and occurred three times within the same year, has lasted fewer than 2 weeks but occurred a lot more than three times in the same year, or has lasted more than 2 weeks and occurred fewer than 3 times in a year.

Functionally Limiting Needs

This means a definite reduction of the activities of daily living or definite problems in maintaining social functioning or difficulty in completing tasks in a timely fashion due to the inability to concentrate or the ability to be persistent.

After an application is received, Social Security usually sends form 4814-F5 to the applicant's physician for completion and submission. Ideally, the physician and the client should fill it out together so nothing is overlooked. This cannot be stressed enough—the objective is to prove that for whatever reason the individual is no longer able to work, and every piece of documented evidence is helpful.

Areas that should not be forgotten are disabling depression, drug and alcohol addiction and the efforts to seek rehabilitative treatment, and the often disabling effects of HIV/AIDS-related medications. If any of these conditions exist, document them, have administrators at work and at rehabilitative programs write letters validating the conditions, and submit the letters with the form. Persistence can make a difference. Local Social Security officers are there to help, so don't give up easily; phone them, visit them, and make them your ally.

According to a study conducted by the Orphan Project in New York City, "the combined assistance from SSI, rental assistance, food, nutrition and transportation programs, could total more than $1,900 per month for a parent with AIDS and two children" (Levine & Stein, 1994, p. 29), a sum not to be sneezed at. Every effort needs to be made to provide as much financial support and security as possible. The affected family has more than enough anxiety without the additional burden of worrying whether the rent will be paid or that there will be food on the table.

Family planning and safer sex involve the most intimate and private area of our lives. Both are subjects all too frequently not discussed with sexual partners. They are affected by culture, religion, taboos, machismo, expectations, abuse, and livelihoods and can result in pregnancy and ultimately in death.

FAMILY PLANNING AND SAFER SEX

During the past several decades, much of the world has recognized the need for family planning as our globally exploding population growth has eaten into world economies and natural resources. Family planning clinics can now be found in many countries and would seem to be a natural place to provide education on STDs and HIV/AIDS. However, their mission is to prevent pregnancy or to provide, as it is popularly referred to, fertility control.

Family planning programs seek and promote ever more "secure" methods of family planning. And secure methods mean long-acting, relatively foolproof procedures which—unlike the condom—may not require partner cooperation, and can be administered in a health care setting, and include sterilization, intrauterine devices (IUD's), injectable contraceptives or implants—none of which protect against HIV. (de Selincourt, 1994, p. 6)

Preventing the Transmission of HIV

As countries report increasing numbers of HIV-infected citizens, it behooves family planning organizations and other reproductive health services to, at the very least, provide HIV prevention information. In some countries such as Kenya, the integration of family planning and HIV education is already occurring (de Selincourt, 1994), and it is hoped that similar programs will expand worldwide.

We know latex condoms do provide safer sex, but in many countries the use of condoms may have to be negotiated according to the prevailing sexual and behavioral attitudes of men. These attitudes and behaviors are influenced by age, culture, education, HIV/AIDS knowledge, machismo, substance use, cultural acceptance of male promiscuity, and women still being regarded as second-class citizens with little or no choice as to how and when they participate in sexual intercourse.

NEGOTIATING SAFER SEX

For a woman, knowing how to negotiate the use of condoms may mean the difference between life and death, so here are some things that the health professional can teach clients.

Developing Negotiating Skills

The first thing is to feel comfortable talking about one's own body with one's partner. This is something that often feels embarrassing and confusing, particularly if the woman was brought up to feel that her task was to provide pleasure to her partner and that her own needs were of less importance. Women have the right to receive pleasure, but most of all women should have the right to be safe. Conversations regarding sex are more productive when they are held in a neutral place (not the bedroom or back seat of a car when the libido is probably going to get in the way) and when both people are relaxed and not sexually aroused. Conversations should not be in a public place or when one is tired, angry, drunk, or stoned.

Conversation can be started in a general way, possibly by discussing a newspaper article, television presentation, or an HIV/AIDS brochure available from any Health and Rehabilitative Service program, libraries, and community-based HIV/AIDS programs. This provides an opportunity to find out who knows what and to identify each individual's beliefs and attitudes regarding HIV/AIDS. Conversation gradually needs to become as intimate as possible; being safe means talking as honestly as possible before doing anything. Finding sexual words that are understandable, descriptive, and inoffensive to each partner is an art in itself. A helpful way to negotiate the language to be used is to have each partner write down a list of acceptable and unacceptable words, discuss each other's list, and agree on what is all right and what is not.

Effectively Using a Condom

No sex at all is the only safe sex, and no protection should equal no sex. Condom use is a safer but not entirely foolproof method. Condoms should be used for all new relationships when the partnership is not monogamous, when one partner is found to be infected, or when both partners are infected as this provides protection against the transmission of other diseases. Condoms should be used for vaginal, anal, and oral sex, every time. Many men resist the whole idea of condoms, stating that the use of condoms "prevents spontaneity," "they are uncomfortable," "they are itchy," "they reduce sensitivity," or the perennial "it's unnecessary because we love each other."

Using a condom does not have to disrupt sex if it is readily accessible and if using one becomes a normal and fun part of foreplay. There are many different types available, varying in price, flavor, shape, and size. Condoms must be made from latex, which is nonporous and therefore cannot transmit diseases. Skin condoms made from animal membranes are porous and potentially lethal. Condoms may be bought nonlubricated or lubricated with a spermicide such as Nonoxynol-9 or a water-based lubricant. Do remember that Nonoxynol-9 is not for everybody. Some people are either sensitive or allergic to it. Sensitive or allergic reactions can lead to the development of irritation and ulcers in the vaginal wall, causing discomfort and more risk for the transmission of other STDs. To find out if there is any sensitivity, suggest that the client spread a little Nonoxynol-9 on the arm. If there is redness or irritation, the Nonoxynol-9 should not be used. Other types of water-based lubricants such as K-Y Jelly can be used.

Professionals should be prepared to instruct clients on how to use condoms. If the client is unfamiliar with putting on a condom, he or she should practice first. Open the packet carefully. Remember that long fingernails and jewelry can tear a condom. Don't unroll a condom when it comes out of the packet as it will become useless! Squeeze the tip of the condom to release any trapped air and put some water-based lubricant into the nipple-shaped teat that holds the semen after the partner's ejaculation. Don't be afraid to improve the technique by trying it out on a large carrot, cucumber, banana, or sex toy such as a vibrator. Practice does make perfect! When everything is ready and the mood is right, hold the rolled-up condom at the tip of the erect penis with one hand and with the other unroll the condom down to the base of the penis, leaving either the nipple, or if there is no nipple about half inch of condom, free to receive the semen. After sex, withdrawal should occur before the penis goes limp, as otherwise the condom may come off, spilling semen into the vagina or anus. Hold the condom around the base of the penis during withdrawal so that spillage is prevented.

FEMALE CONDOMS OR FEMIDOMS

Female condoms have been available in Europe for several years and are now becoming obtainable in the United States. Their biggest advantages are the control and power that they give women to protect themselves and that they can be inserted by oneself or with assistance from a partner rather than by a health professional.

The most popular one is a pouch that lines the vagina and is anchored by two flexible rings, one of which is inserted into the vagina and the other of which stays outside. Many of us tend to ignore package instructions, but study the diagram, read the directions, and have a practice run. Female condoms can be removed immediately, but can be inserted ahead of time—a definite plus as it takes care of the spontaneity issue. They are thinner than male condoms as they are made out of polyurethane and therefore feel more natural for both partners. They are resistant to the effects of oil-based lubricants, and because the labia and urethra are covered, lessen the potential for receiving any STDs.

Unfortunately, some women dislike putting any form of contraceptive into their vagina and so will not use this kind of barrier protection. Female condoms are also not cheap, which will put them out of the reach of the most needy group, the economically disadvantaged. It is hoped that as they become more available the cost will lessen.

Remember, no condom is 100% reliable and that other ways to enjoy sex include talking about sex and sharing fantasies; stroking and nibbling nipples, fingers, hands, toes, and ear lobes; massaging, cuddling, hugging, and stroking; kissing inner thighs, behind the knees, palms, inner elbows, shoulders, and base of the neck; masturbation of self; masturbation of one's partner; and using sex toys (however, they should never be shared with others without first washing them thoroughly).

In real life, do remember that there are many women who are not able to insist on their partners using a condom because they fear being physically or emotionally abused. This is true particularly when the women are poor or live in countries where they are considered to be second class citizens without rights. Indeed, their fears may be well justified. They are in a true dilemma of putting their lives at risk either for injury or for HIV infection. Until there are effective, practical, and female-controlled barrier protections readily and cheaply available to all women, many women will continue to play Russian roulette with their lives. According to Dr. Hitchcock from NIAID, a barrier method would ideally be colorless, odorless, and tasteless; stable (not influenced by changes in the temperature); inexpensive;

easy to use; active immediately and for the duration of sexual intercourse; available without a prescription; and not disruptive to the vaginal flora (Denison, 1993). Developing safer sex strategies can happen if there is support, understanding, and determination. Lori Heise of the Center for Women's Global Leadership in New York tells the story "of sex workers in Nigeria who organized themselves and agreed that they would all double their prices on the same day, at the same time and not undercut each other. In that way, they could all afford to turn down customers who refused to wear a condom" (Denison, 1993, p. 3).

Women are being infected with HIV in many ways, but at least half the transmission rate is in some way drug related. Included in this category are women who do not use drugs but who are infected by a drug-using HIV-infected sex partner (Osborn, 1991).

DRUG REHABILITATION

Those who are already addicted to drugs may also become alcoholics. This lifestyle frequently causes extreme mobility, moving from place to place with no fixed address, which makes locating, intervention, and support extraordinarily challenging! Location and effective follow-up will be affected by family support systems, language barriers, cultural barriers, and lifestyles.

For the health care professional to provide intervention, it is necessary to have compassion, determination, an understanding of the street language of drugs, and a respect for confidentiality; to be a good and innovative communicator; and to know the community resources. Effective intervention can only be based on need, motivation, and trust. Developing trust takes time; energy; honesty; knowledge of HIV; a genuine desire to help; an understanding of social, cultural, and economic issues; and a recognition that behavioral changes are never easy and frequently resemble a roller coaster ride.

HIV/AIDS risk-related behaviors, like all behaviors, are tied to every part of our lives. Drug dealing may be the base for financial stability, a roof over one's head, and food for the kids. Low self-esteem, little validation, a lifetime of powerlessness, social support from one's own peer group for unsafe behaviors, and little or no available rehabilitation resources all contribute to maintaining the status quo and continuance of potentially harmful outcomes. Women of color are at a particular risk as their poverty rate is more than double that of White women, causing women of color to suffer from substandard or no housing, insufficient food and clothing, and inadequate access to health services.

Empowerment for women revolves around a client–counselor relationship based on collaboration, trust, the sharing of power, genuineness, mutual respect, open communication, and informality (Gutierrez, 1990). Community education and committed community support may be the best way to develop personal responsibility and empowerment, validation, and self-esteem, particularly using as role models those who have walked the path of chemical addiction and who have chosen to recover. Behavioral modification messages are often understood better when they are delivered by individuals with whom we identify and who speak and sound and behave similarly to us.

A group of women whose HIV/AIDS issues are infrequently addressed are those who are older, above the age of 55. Indeed, a search of the relevant literature turned up absolutely nothing. Although little is known about this population, it should not be forgotten.

OLDER WOMEN AND HIV/AIDS

Before 1985 and the introduction of strict guidelines for the collection of blood and tissue, a number of older people were infected by HIV-contaminated blood during surgical procedures. Diagnosis was often made late, support systems were frequently weak, and medical intervention was poor because the majority of physicians who look after elderly persons are neither infectious disease specialists nor knowledgeable regarding diagnosis, care, and treatment for HIV.

Today, at-risk older individuals can be those whose first marriage was for many years and who then find themselves single and looking for a partner. That in itself has its share of hazards, but an older woman rarely knows much about condom use and is unlikely to jeopardize a relationship with a man by either asking about his past or suggesting that he use a condom.

Others at risk are women whose spouses do not maintain monogamous relationships, women involved with illegal substances, women whose partners abuse chemical substances, and women who have multiple sexual partners. These are difficult subjects to discuss with anyone and are usually shrouded in shame, blame, guilt, and fear.

Dr. Marcia Ory, the chief of social science research at the National Institute of Aging in Bethesda, Maryland, has suggested that because a woman's uterine lining becomes thinner as she ages, older women may be more susceptible to the AIDS virus. Also, as women grow older, immune systems may weaken, which could cause the virus to travel faster (Kellerman, 1994).

If an older person presents signs and symptoms that sound like HIV, don't hesitate to encourage them to go to see an infectious disease specialist, but do remember to provide them with a lot of ongoing support related to their age, otherwise its relevancy will be lost.

Help family members to help infected persons by providing accurate information and education, and if it is possible, find or start a support group to assist them. Most support groups are for younger people and may be uncomfortable for the older person who is often embarrassed to talk about HIV/AIDS and will be confronting different issues than the younger person.

Throughout the country, grandmothers whose daughters have died of AIDS are looking after infected children; some are infected themselves. It has taken some time, but they have now banded together as a group and share their sorrows and triumphs together at weekly meetings; bring in speakers on the medical, psychosocial, spiritual, and child care dimensions of HIV; assist with clothes and food banks; maintain a daily telephone call-around to the homebound; speak in the community; take the HIV message to their churches; and generally provide nonjudgmental, loving support to anyone who needs it.

It is most important to not forget older persons. We do a dreadful disservice to them if we allow either them or ourselves to believe that it cannot happen to them. Support groups can provide a wonderful opportunity for people to communicate and enhance their lives and to develop coping strategies that encourage them to live with this retrovirus called HIV.

SUPPORT GROUPS FOR WOMEN

Early support groups were male oriented and male attended as that population was the first in the United States to manifest HIV/AIDS. As women became increasingly affected and infected, the need for women's support groups became more apparent. Women's groups can now be found in many metropolitan areas. The following paragraphs suggest some things to consider if you do not have one in your area, want to start one, and are wondering how to begin.

Market Survey

There is no point in starting a group if one isn't needed! Telephone local AIDS organizations and find out if they offer a women's group. If they do not, ask if they would be willing to refer to you women who ask for one. Contact organizations and individuals who serve PWAs such as hospitals, primary care clinics, hospices, churches, synagogues, public health departments, physicians, social workers, psychologists, dentists, and discharge planners; explain your intentions; and ask if they would refer their female clients to you.

When you have decided that there is a need, and the time and location is established, send announcements to possible participants, local newspapers' "Coming Events" calendars, church and synagogue bulletin boards, local AIDS organizations, radio and television stations as a public service announcement, health professionals, your United Way agency, and other organizations who have expressed an interest.

Time and Location

Many working people prefer a weekday evening from 6:30 to 8:00 P.M. If there are children who need a sitter, a family member is often available in the evening. Remember that nothing is set in stone. Days and times can always be changed to suit the participants' needs.

The location should be central, comfortable, wheelchair accessible, and handicapped friendly, including the restroom. The room should be private as confidentiality is an integral part of establishing trust.

The Facilitator

Whoever runs the group should have most of the following talents and resources: committed for the long haul, knowledgeable regarding women's issues and HIV, nonjudgmental, good sense of humor, flexible, empathetic without pity, reasonably goal oriented, access to outside speakers; knowledgeable regarding local community resources, leadership ability, the skills to diffuse acrimony and anger, the recognition that there are not always solutions, and the capacity to maintain a positive healthy attitude.

Setting Up the Room

Include a sign-up sheet and pen (Ask for the name and phone number of the participant, who may or may not wish to give either—don't push it initially. As trust builds, information is more forthcoming.); marker pens and name labels (use first names only); chairs set in a circle; boxes of tissues; regular and decaffeinated coffee; tea; soft drinks; sweetener and milk; disposable cups, plates, and utensils; cookies, cakes, and so forth; VCR and tape player; flip chart or blackboard; and a table for handouts. Handouts can include current research material, medication protocols available locally, national and local HIV/AIDS hotline numbers, a list of local resources, brochures on healthy nutrition, SSI booklets from the Social Security Administration, and uplifting poems and articles. The list is endless, and material is usually free and readily available from public health departments, HIV/AIDS organizations, the state AIDS hotlines, National Clinical Trials Information Service (1-800-874-2572), and the National AIDS Clearing House (1-800-358-9295). The latter are but two of the many 800 numbers available, and one resource invariably leads to another.

General Format

You may choose to make the groups ongoing (If so, make certain you have a backup facilitator; you will need a break!) or for periods of 6, 8, or 10 weeks, and so forth. Groups can develop their own format, shaped by the participants' needs, or follow a more structured program. A little of each seems to work the best. As the group progresses, you will discover the most satisfactory formula to follow and the most needed subject matter to cover.

Group Size

When groups number more than 15 persons, they become unwieldy, with the danger of individual needs becoming lost in the crowd. At that point, it may be possible to divide the group and have two, or you may find that you don't mind how large it is.

Rules of the Road

A few simple rules that are identified at the beginning of each meeting encourage harmony, individual participation, and positive outcomes. Again, these are only suggestions, and you may prefer to have no rules or a totally different list from these. What has worked for me includes identifying the meaning, importance, and trust issues surrounding confidentiality; having one person speak at a time and for no longer than 3 minutes (this rarely works but gives one an opportunity to call a halt when someone begins to monopolize, and someone usually does); allowing no comparisons of situations as it becomes an "I'm worse off than you are, therefore you cannot possible understand me" situation; listening, without interruption, to each other; avoiding giving unsolicited advice; exchanging telephone numbers only, unless you don't mind unexpected, possibly disruptive visits to your home; starting on time, otherwise latecomers miss vital parts or the group has to return to the beginning; finishing on time; remembering that drinking, illegal drug use, and driving do not mix; not forbidding smoking unless by state law, but allowing it in designated areas only; not allowing illegal drugs and alcohol on the premises; welcoming donations for refreshments; helping to tidy the room before leaving; parking cars in a well-lighted area; and leaving together.

Introductions and Expectations

Name tags help people to identify each other. At the beginning of each session, have each person introduce him- or herself and ask them to say why they are here and what they hope to receive from the group. Their expectations can be written on the flip chart, which then provides a basic road map to follow. These expectations can be pinned up around the room at each session.

Content of the Sessions

The sky's the limit and content will depend on the group's needs, but it could include basic HIV/AIDS education and information; information on condom use; needle cleaning and needle-exchange programs; assertiveness training; healthy lifestyles through exercise and nutrition; foster parenting; child care; Social Security, SSI, and SSDI; spiritual issues; advance directives, living wills, wills, and personal power of attorney; stress management; positive decision making; living positively; massage therapy; guided imagery and visualization; research medications and protocols; community resources; HIV/AIDS and pregnancy; family planning; time management versus procrastination; advocacy; management and care of HIV-infected children; and dealing with anger, guilt, and so forth. Use outside speakers who are able to discuss their own areas of expertise in a language that is comprehensive and enjoyable.

Outside Speakers

Some suggestions for outside speakers are a physician expert in HIV issues, social worker, discharge planner, drug company representative, panel of HIV-positive (HIV+) individuals, pastoral counselor, Social Security Administration representative, massage therapist, attorney, panel representing HIV/AIDS organizations, substance abuse counselor, nutritionist, children's advocate, pediatric nurse, and foster parent.

Support groups are a wonderful way to develop empowerment, cohesiveness, education, friendship, resources, sharing, balance, commitment, and a sense of belonging. Encourage your group members to maintain positive outlooks and healthy lifestyles. The long-term effect of a well-run group can be nothing short of miraculous. Enjoy!

The other part of this chapter addresses children's issues, including children's needs when they and their parents are HIV+, children who lose a sibling to HIV, adolescence and HIV, grandparents who face the loss of their present and future, and foster parents caring for HIV-infected children.

THE HIV+ FAMILY

One of the tragedies of HIV is the increasing rate of infection among children and adolescents. In the latter part of this century, sub-Saharan Africa witnessed a decrease in its infant and childhood deaths as a result of hard-won improvements in the delivery of health care to children. In April 1994, the U.S. Bureau of the Census predicted "that unless there was a sharp slowing in the rate of [HIV] infection in these countries, childhood mortality rates would triple by the year 2010" (Holmes, 1994, p. 11).

In the United States, as HIV infection continues to rise among young women of childbearing age, so too does the consequent infection rate in babies. Whatever should happen in the way of preventive vaccines or curative medications, by the year 2000 there will be an unknown number of infected and affected orphaned children from the results of AIDS. Of these children, a disproportionate number will be children of color or of Hispanic origin. As a nation, health care providers, and individuals, it behooves us to address the complex, multigenerational issues of children with HIV/AIDS sooner rather than later.

CHILDREN AND HIV

Transmission

Transmission occurs in approximately 25% of perinatally exposed infants. However, all exposed infants "will suffer the consequences of being born into a family in which one or more adult is infected with HIV" (U.S. Department of Health and Human Services, 1994, p. 81). Transmission occurs either in utero (i.e., during pregnancy) or intrapartum (i.e., at the time of birth). Rarely babies may be infected by their infected mother's breast milk. Long-term surviving children are those who have the benefits of early diagnosis and aggressive, supportive, and HIV-specific treatment.

Signs and Symptoms of HIV Infection in Babies

Symptoms of HIV infection in babies include the following: swelling in the lymph glands in the neck, under the arms, and in the diaper area; swollen belly, sometimes with diarrhea (frequent loose, watery bowel movements); itchy skin rashes; frequent lung infections (pneumonia); frequent ear and sinus infections;

problems with gaining weight or growth (failure to thrive); inability to do the kinds of things healthy babies do (such as sitting alone, crawling, walking); and crankiness, irritability, and constant crying.

Do remember that the client should immediately report any of these symptoms or other changes to the doctor.

Diagnosis

The U.S. Department of Health and Human Services (1994) in its 1994 clinical practice guidelines for HIV recommended that the following steps be taken:

- *All infants born to HIV-infected mothers should be monitored to determine HIV status.*
- *In the HIV-exposed infant under 18 months of age, use of virus culture or polymerase chain reaction is the preferred method for diagnosis of HIV infection. If these tests are not available, P24 antigen assays should be used for diagnosis. One or more of these HIV-specific tests should be done as soon as possible after 1 month of age and if negative should be repeated between 3 and 6 months of age. Infants with negative diagnostic tests at 6 months of age should have an HIV antibody test (enzyme-linked immunosorbent assay, or ELISA) performed at 15 and 18 months of age to document HIV infection status.*
- *In the child over 18 months of age, testing for antibody to HIV using the standard ELISA test with an approved confirmatory test is sufficient for diagnosis of HIV.*

Treatment

Treatment for young children is under continuing modification as more is understood about the progression of the virus in children. Current methods are antiretroviral therapy administered either because of the presenting symptoms of HIV infection or because of lowered CD4 counts, frequent monitoring, neurologic testing, supportive care, tuberculosis screening, nutritional supplementations, and immunization for certain childhood diseases.

Treatment is expensive and because of the expense will not be available to many of the world's infected children. Treatment may mean pain and side effects from medication, separation from a parent, confusion, and bewilderment. Young children cannot easily communicate their needs and, at a time of illness, are often surrounded by adults who may inflict all kinds of demands on them, further adding to their distress. It is up to us to try and make their world a little safer and more secure. Their practical living needs are every bit as important as their medication protocols.

Practical Needs of Young Children

Regardless of what is done medically, children who are born to HIV-infected mothers are almost certainly going to lose that parent to an early death. This takes away the most important person in that infant's life. Indeed, all children need and deserve love, attention, and care and already may be unwanted by their natural parents or possibly by their adoptive parents because of their seropositivity. It is imperative that somehow a way is found to provide and maintain stable and sustained relationships in places of safety, preferably within the family system, by using more creative and innovative methods of support such as coparenting.

Coparenting

Coparenting is a new option for foster care relationships that provides the support these children need within a new framework of foster care provision that works in situations in which the parents are still alive, but may either be having difficulty coping with the diagnosed child or be dealing with their own HIV status. Through coparenting, agreements are reached whereby birth parents and foster parents share responsibility for caring for the child, such as by taking care of the child for 3 days on an alternating basis. This system provides a transition for the child when a parent dies by giving the child two homes in which he or she is comfortable, in turn easing the blow of losing a parent or parents.

This model can also help those children who are not HIV+, whose parents are dying, and who need both respite care from a traumatic and difficult situation and later stability and support from an already known family. This, of course, will only work if legal arrangements are made before the death of the parent or parents occurs.

Foster parenting fills a desperately needed gap for those children who, for whatever reason, cannot live in their biological family home.

Foster Parenting

Foster parents can be other family members or other willing families. Foster parents must, before committing to welcoming an HIV-infected child into their home, think about the meaning of this kind of commitment. They must remember that at least one of the child's parents will almost certainly die; that there is continuing medical treatment to follow; that the child may have a series of illnesses requiring extra care, love, and support; and that eventually the child will also die. Prospective foster and adoptive parents need to project the course of care through to its ultimate end. HIV-infected children may rapidly become seriously ill, deteriorate quickly, and die unexpectedly. Foster and adoptive parents need to know their own coping skills at times of crisis and loss and must be in good health themselves. None of the above is said to deter but as a reminder that this kind of involvement will have laughter, tears, joy, and sorrow.

Foster parents need to be comfortable and educated regarding the prevention of HIV transmission; the signs and symptoms of HIV and the more common opportunistic infections associated with full-blown AIDS; universal precautions; the availability of HIV testing; day care; school issues; working with health and rehabilitative services, which can be a bureaucratic jungle; issues of the child's biological family; support services; and community resources.

Ideally, foster parents and biological parents should be able to play an interactive role in the child's care, with thoughtful, wise decisions made through discussion and agreement. Sadly, because of inadequate preparation, children may be passed from the natural family to a group home to a foster home to an adoptive home and then, if the adoptive family finds that the child is more than they can handle emotionally or physically, the cycle will start all over again. It is hard to imagine how difficult this must be for the child.

Adequate and intensive counseling at the very beginning, before the child leaves his or her natural home, could change a potentially negative outcome to a very positive event. Not only is this the best solution for the child, but parents will know that their child will be loved, comforted, nurtured, and cherished.

Becoming a Foster Parent

There is a formal process that may be slightly different in each state; however, the counselor should be aware of the general guidelines. Applicants contact the local child welfare agent and state that they would like to become foster parents; a social worker will then make a visit to the home to evaluate how the home is kept, if there is adequate space for a foster child or children, and that it meets minimum standards for health and safety such as having functioning fire extinguishers, smoke detectors, and separate beds for each foster child. There may be a request for a statement from the applicant's physician concerning the foster parents' health and they may have to be tested for certain communicable diseases such as tuberculosis (Gilsenan, 1994, p. 244). A background check is initiated on all adult family members, and if there are any records of complaints or convictions involving child abuse or neglect, the applicant will be turned down as a foster parent.

Foster parenting does not necessarily mean that individuals have to be married or nonworking. Indeed, a number of foster parents caring for children with HIV are single women. They have found this kind of care incredibly emotionally rewarding.

Training is available to the foster parent that helps with the physical and emotional needs of the child and with understanding the bureaucratic and legal process. There should be HIV-specific education offered and suggestions regarding the availability of additional support and resources. A stipend is paid for each child but is barely adequate, so foster parents will give a lot because of desire and love.

The applicant should remember that the child may not stay forever and that, under the law, a foster parent's rights are exceedingly limited. Usually, the child remains in the custody of the state and can therefore be moved from the home at any time. However, with the specific needs of these particular children, there is a good chance that they will stay with the foster parents until death occurs. Encourage people who want to be foster parents and help them to work through the red tape—these kids really need them.

Adoption is another protective system that offers far more legal guarantees than foster parenting.

ADOPTION OF AFFECTED AND INFECTED CHILDREN

Adopting any child can be a lengthy and frustrating process. Adopting an HIV-infected child or children is a life event that needs to be carefully considered. This youngster is one who will eventually become ill, and whose death, at the present time, is almost certain. Illness can cause many disruptions and, unless the adopting family is truly focused by their desire to make this loving commitment, it may place the entire family into chaos, fear, anger, denial, and distress. However, the adoptive parents that I have had the privilege to know have found inner resources of strength to cope with every crisis cheerfully and courageously and say that the love that is given to them by the children is a payment that cannot be quantified.

Anyone can be adopted as the child of someone else regardless of their age. Relatives, including stepparents, can adopt a child, and when this is possible, this is a wonderful way to go as it keeps children within a system and culture already known to them. Every state allows parents to place a child or children with a relative, and in some states parents can let nonrelatives adopt their child.

The most important factor is that these arrangements should be made before the death of the parents if they are to be effective and to save the youngster from even further trauma. Talking about such intensely emotional issues with parents is not easy and requires patience, compassion, understanding of the particular family system, and perseverance. If possible, try to keep siblings together as their lives are probably already full of bewilderment and confusion.

Legal Steps in an Adoption

The following are very brief guidelines for adoption, and each state may be a little different both in adoption proceedings and issues of HIV. Local HIV agencies and attorneys should be able to suggest local resources. There may be an attorney willing to help with this process for a nominal fee or no fee at all.

Notice. This is given to everyone legally interested in the case, excluding the child.

Petition. The adopting parents must formally apply to the court for permission to adopt the child.

Written consent. The natural parents of the child must authorize in writing their agreement to the adoption of the child. This goes with the petition.

Hearing. A court hearing, which is confidential, occurs in which the qualifications of the adopting parents are examined. The petition will then be granted or denied.

Probation. There is usually a period of supervision by a state agency after the adoption to see that everyone can adapt happily to one another. The adoption becomes final only after the period of supervision is completed.

Birth certificate. A new birth certificate will be issued, giving a new family name. The old birth certificate is sealed and filed. It is usually not available unless a court order is obtained.

Finding a Child

State-licensed adoption agencies should help. They will have rules and regulations that are developed by state laws, and adopting parents must abide by those laws. Local community-based HIV/AIDS agencies and public health programs should also be able to help, so don't hesitate to call on them.

Like foster parents, adoptive parents should be well versed in HIV/AIDS transmission, symptoms, and treatment; health care delivery systems; confidentiality issues; local resources; financial aid; scholastic education; issues surrounding loss; external support systems; and support systems within the family. Adoption requires special and dedicated people and gives a child things that are irreplaceable—support, security, and love at that child's most needy time.

Another area that the counselor needs to be aware of is child care centers and HIV-infected children in group settings. Group settings include church and temple nurseries, private day care, prekindergarten, kindergarten, and migrant care.

The goal is to remember that it is really important that infected and affected children be treated as normally as possible. Sadly, past experience tells us that this is not always the case. Newspaper headlines have told the nation of infected children being isolated in school settings, families being discriminated against, homes being burnt, and so on. As the public becomes more knowledgeable regarding HIV, it is to be hoped that the stigmas attached to the disease will not only lessen, but disappear. This is still not the case. However, by taking some simple steps parental and employee fears can be reduced, and all children can receive care in a safe, secure, and friendly environment.

GUIDELINES FOR GROUP CHILD CARE SETTINGS*

In many child care settings, whether employees are aware or not, there may well be an infected child. Education and training for employees is essential to reduce their fears and to develop positive outcomes.

Basic Education

An introduction to HIV/AIDS and other infectious diseases, given in simple language and delivered in an informal atmosphere, encourages the participants to ask questions and discuss their concerns. No question is silly if the answer is not known.

Universal Precautions

Universal precautions remind us that everyone should be treated as if they are infected. When anyone cuts themselves or spills blood, latex disposable gloves should be worn to avoid any contact with blood or bodily fluids containing the blood. Use paper towels and a disinfectant to wipe up spills, including those that spill onto the floor. Don't use a mop. Dispose of the gloves and paper towels by putting them into a sealed plastic bag and then into an outside trash container.

Latex Gloves

Gloves need not be used to wipe up bodily fluids in which blood is not visible. These fluids include urine, tears, nasal discharge, saliva, stools, and vomit. Hands must be washed after handling any bodily fluid. Gloves should be used once and then disposed of properly.

*Some of this material was adapted from *A Staff Manual About AIDS and HIV Infection for Child Care Centers* (Wise, 1993).

Washing Hands

Good hand washing saves lives and prevents the transmission of a variety of diseases. Staff and children should wash hands before eating, feeding, or handling food; after toileting or diapering; before and after giving first aid; after wiping noses, mouths, bottoms, and sores; after cleaning surfaces soiled with bodily fluids (blood, mucous, vomit); before giving medicine; and after taking off disposable gloves. Staff who have hands that are dry, chapped, cracked, or sore should wear disposable gloves for diapering and for handling strong cleansers. Use mild soap for hand washing and regularly apply a hand lotion. If the cracks and sores persist, the employee should seek medical advice.

Disinfectant Solution

A cheap and effective disinfectant is made by mixing 1 gallon of water with ¼ quarter cup of bleach. Fill empty spray containers with the mixed solution, and have them clearly labeled and easily available.

Supplies

Supplies are useless unless they are kept in easily accessible and known places. Supplies need to be indoors, outdoors, and on transportation buses. One innovative center has adapted large nail aprons bought in a hardware store. Teachers and helpers wear them in the playground. The pockets have a supply of paper towels, latex gloves, and a small first aid kit. They are ready for any emergency!

Glove dispensers and glove canisters are available from a variety of suppliers. They have belt clips or double-faced velcro and can be worn out of doors; containers can be wall mounted inside and outside.

Demonstration

The educator should physically demonstrate where products are, how they should be used, how to dispose of them, and where the dumpster is. Fear arises when we don't know how to do things. This is one fear that shouldn't arise!

Teaching the Children

Very small children can be taught how germs are spread and how to protect themselves. They need to know that when they cut themselves, the wound should be immediately cleaned and covered; they should not remove scabs as scabs help healing and prevent further bleeding; they should not share toothbrushes or drinking mugs; they should never ever bite another person; they should cover their nose and mouth when they sneeze and cough; they should report a cut or injury of any kind to themselves or to their friends to their teacher as soon as possible; and washing their hands can prevent the spread of germs.

Confidentiality and Discrimination Issues

Parents or guardians can be asked if their child is HIV+, but they have the right not to say. Disclosure can be both positive and negative. It may increase social support, encourage other family members to be tested, and permit enhanced entitlement benefits. On the negative side, disclosure may open a virtual Pandora's box of issues that could include discrimination to parents, guardians, and the child; loss of child custody; loss of employment; reduction or cessation of health benefits; rejection by a potential employer, significant other, or religious and public school system.

If the parent does say that the child is HIV+, the family's rights should be carefully protected, and the information kept private. The only people who need to know the child's status are the director, the health care coordinator, and the child's immediate supervisor.

Children who are HIV+ cannot be refused admission to group settings for children if these centers are receiving federal or state funds. Private organizations should also not discriminate but have been known to refuse children whom they either know or suspect are HIV+. Education is the way to change these attitudes!

Further Staff Education

Staff education should include sensitivity training. A powerful exercise is to have individuals imagine what it would be like to have a child who is HIV+ and the questions and feelings this would create: "Would I tell?" "Who would I tell?" "What does this mean to my family?" "Am I positive?" "What about the other kids?" and so forth. Personalizing the possibility is a way of letting people feel in their hearts rather than think in their heads.

Have a hospice employee come in and talk to staff about the possible course of a terminal illness; the needs of the child, family, and staff; and death, grief, and bereavement. Everyone grieves when a child dies. Having a bereavement counselor identify the grief process and suggest intervention strategies to assist with grief work validates the child's life and the feelings of those who cared for that child. Grief and bereavement are discussed further in chapter 9.

Parent–Guardian Involvement

Parents, foster parents, and guardians need to be an integral part of the child's care. This is a time when they need support, compassion, and empathy. Other things may be occurring in their lives that may be equally tumultuous. Any way that they can be helped by child care centers will relieve some of their anxiety and fears and will give them a little more energy to deal with other life issues.

THE SICK CHILD

Children first and foremost are children and should be treated as such. All too often, when adults know that a child has a terminal illness they treat the child differently. Frequently, children do not know their diagnosis, or if they do or think they do, they are discouraged from talking about it. Their bodies are treated to many indignities, some of which are extraordinarily painful, while they are being assured that "this won't hurt" or being exhorted to "be a man." Parents and health professionals tend to treat them as younger than they actually are when the opposite seems to be true—they appear to grow up emotionally at an accelerated pace. Adults try to protect them, and children are adept at seeing through this. Children should be treated as normally as possible in what, for them, is an increasingly changing world. Children need to play, and it does adults a lot of good to play right along with them. Children, either at home or in a medical institution, can enhance their lives through play. Play gives them an opportunity to express their feelings emotionally when they may not be able to do so verbally. HIV-infected children may be facing the loss of their entire family system—parents, grandparents, brothers, and sisters—which will irreparably change their lives forever.

Playing with Kids

Play helps to establish trust; identify unspoken questions; provide peer support systems; distraction from painful events; nonverbal communication; normal emotional development; reveal hostile and angry feelings; develop coping skills; interpret the progression of disease; encourage laughter and joy; and reinforce safety and security.

Play materials. Play materials include coloring books, blank paper, loads of different colored crayons, toys of choice, cuddly toys, musical instruments, puppets, dolls, or whatever is the favorite comforter.

Puppets and dolls are wonderful tools not only to bring out negative feelings, but also to teach a child about medical procedures that will occur. When my youngest daughter was 5 years old, she had to have a heart catheterization. In the 1960s, the process was lengthy (4–5 hours), a very modest sedative was given, and she was not only in a hospital unknown to her but was in another country with unknown people. The night before the procedure, the "cath" team came to her bedside with a puppet surgically dressed and capped. In simple but direct and honest language, they introduced themselves, played with her big doll, and then told her about the procedure using the puppet. They were clear about their expectations of her. She promptly fell in love with the gorgeous South African, 6-foot, 2-inch, male leader of the team, who promised to come back and say good night to her, which he did. The next morning, she was wheeled off to the theater, clutching the puppet, calm and confident, and serenely returned to a wreck of a mother some hours later. She was told that she was the best ever, had followed the instructions faithfully, and hadn't moved an inch. The puppet is still around, bashed and battered but a reminder of how explanations can prevent unnecessary anxiety and promote positive care.

Art therapy. You, the counselor, are not expected to be an art therapist. However, if you are armed with blank paper and many crayons, children will often spontaneously draw at a conscious and subconscious level the events that are happening to them, where they see themselves and their illness in these events, and what their expectations are for their future. By either asking gentle open-ended questions or telling the child what you see in the picture, you may encourage the child to talk his or her own meanings out with you.

Videos, audiocassettes, and other suggestions. Older children may like to make a video of their family life or record the history of the family on audiocassettes. Children who are terminally ill have written books and some wonderful poems about what is happening to them. Some kids love to have a "point-and-shoot" camera and will document their everyday happenings in film and written word.

Humor. Kids usually have a wonderfully slapstick sense of humor. Old Laurel and Hardy movies will often convulse them. Visits by clowns can elicit anything from giggles of mirth to belly laughs. Funny costumes, masks, false noses, and wigs can be highly entertaining. Laughter distracts them from their immediate issues and makes everyone feel better.

Make-A-Wish Foundation. This foundation can make a wish come true for children and their families. This could be a visit to Disney World, the visit of a well-known sports figure to their home or hospital, or a ride in a fire engine—almost anything that the child truly desires. Ask your local Make-A-Wish group and see what they can do.

Camps. There are now several camps throughout the United States who host kids who are HIV-infected. The camps are for 10 days to 2 weeks and provide an enormous opportunity for children to be with their peers in a very upbeat atmosphere. Camp may be the first time that they are able to share the secret of their HIV status and what it has felt like keeping that secret. Camp gives kids the time and place to just be kids. They don't have to be afraid of the external or internal environment; counselors are there to love and listen; children can have fun and share their innermost thoughts in a supportive, dynamic, and loving environment.

Play is about maintaining hope, lifting depression, and celebrating life. Keeping life normal also means that children should continue to attend school.

School

Stimulation and learning are part of the natural cycle of life. School can continue at home and in the hospital. Many larger hospitals have schoolrooms and teachers. Many school boards have a home-bound classroom program. Children should be encouraged to continue their education as it normalizes their lives, keeps them in contact with friends, and prevents them from becoming isolated.

As children become more ill, they tend to slowly go through several stages. Each child is a unique individual and may not manifest any of these stages, so please consider the following guidelines as general markers that may or may not occur.

AWARENESS STAGES

In *The Private Worlds of Dying Children*, there is a statement that "leukemic children acquired factual information about their disease in five stages" (Bluebond-Langer, 1978, p. 166). I believe that in greater or lesser ways all terminally ill children, with whatever disease, become aware in a similar way.

Stage 1

Stage 1 occurs after children have become aware that this is no ordinary illness. They have been poked, prodded, stuck, and x-rayed. This is not a routine trip to the doctor. Because of the stigma attached to HIV, parents may decide not to tell the children that they are HIV+ or the children may be told and in the next breath told to keep it a secret. Already a conspiracy of silence and fear is beginning. At this stage, the children may notice the difference in adult behaviors toward them and may want to talk about the physical changes and things that are being done to them, called the *exhibition of the wounds* (Bluebond-Langer, 1978). Children can be very explicit about who did what, when, and how, and they don't pull any punches as to who hurt and who did not.

Stage 2

Stage 2 is a knowledge-gathering time when children collect information about their medical care and treatment, particularly from other HIV-infected children. Their belief is that they are licking this thing and getting better. HIV is a roller coaster of a disease, so that one minute a child can appear to be dying and a few days later be feeling fine and certainly not dying. As the use of medications and treatments become more effective and children live longer, children will go in and out of Stage 2.

Stage 3

As time progresses and the children are ill more frequently, they are left more to their own devices, receiving less parental information and support and relying heavily on discussing their symptoms and treatments with their peers.

Stage 4

As children move into a more acute terminal stage, their world shrinks. More time is spent in bed, probably in the hospital, and the realization that death does occur becomes a reality. They are visited less by family, staff, friends, and peers. Steadily they become more isolated as they move toward their death.

Stage 5

Children who are actually dying often either talk about death or refer to death when they are playing. Children no longer speak of long-range plans, never mention growing up, and express feelings of not wasting time. This may be a time of hostility, withdrawal, self-isolation, and abandonment, occurring just when they need as much support as they can get.

Children who are in full-blown AIDS need continuous encouragement and support. Unlike other pediatric terminal illnesses, where only one child is sick and the parents are usually well, these children may come from a home environment that is burdened with other tragedies and disasters. Providing treatment and support needs a team effort, creativity, advocacy, and forbearance.

ADVOCACY

Dying children need health professionals to be advocates for them. There are many, many needs, but the two areas that are often particularly neglected in the care of these special children are pain management and allowing a child to die peacefully.

Pain Management

All sorts of procedures are performed on children, usually without their consent and often without their understanding, and little or nothing is given to prevent pain. As the opportunistic infections of AIDS increase, so does pain. When a child is in pain, it is not good enough to make comforting noises or to undermedicate the pain. Children may need morphine for intractable pain in the same way that an adult does. If a young patient of yours is in pain, discuss it with the child's physician and be persistent until something adequate is done. Pain assessment can be made by listening to the child's description of the pain; watching his or her behaviors and mobility, that is, does he or she grimace and cry out? Is he or she able to move easily without discomfort? Is he or she sleeping all night? Is he or she receiving anything for pain? There is a Happy–Sad Face scale that ranges from 0 to 5. *Happy* is zero and means no pain at all and *sad* is 5 and means the worst pain imaginable. This scale allows the child to point to the face that most accurately portrays how he or she is feeling.

Children in pain lose their ability to live well and to be as independent as possible, and we have the skills to make this a very different picture. We should be using them.

Dying

Parents and health professionals, including physicians, find it extraordinarily difficult to let a child die. Consequently, almost until the moment of death it is not uncommon to see a child receiving rehabilitative treatments at a time when comfort and peace should be the goal. As health professionals, we need to recognize what is best for the child, and when it is apparent that curative measures are not working it is not only all right but necessary to allow the child to meet death in as gentle and dignified way as possible.

Death at Home

The death of a child at home is not always possible. Parents and siblings may be acutely afraid of the child dying at home, and symptoms may be alleviated better in the hospital. However, if the child can go home, support this. Call in a hospice team for guidance, support, and family education, and encourage the family to look after the child. This family caring can provide enormous solace and comfort after death has occurred. The family knows that they were there for this beloved youngster and made the final days as rewarding as possible.

CHILDREN WHO LOSE A PARENT
OR A SIBLING TO HIV-RELATED CAUSES

In the HIV-infected and -affected family, it is possible that some siblings are infected and that others are not. Children need to know what is going on when a parent or brother or sister is sick. Too often they are left in the dark, attention is paid to the sick adult or child, and the well child or children feel isolated and confused. How they handle the illness and death of a parent or sibling will very much depend on the level of their knowledge of the illness, how they are treated by the family members, and how involved they are allowed to be with the sick relative.

When one parent dies, it is usually a shattering experience for a child, whatever the child's age. When a youngster faces the loss of multiple family members, the impact will stretch for years into the child's future. The very thought of a parent dying is frightening. These thoughts may be translated into potentially harmful behavior for the child, either self-destructive or injurious to others.

The following example is of a single-parent family including nine children and an HIV-infected mother. The mother lives on welfare and was recently attacked and violently raped in the stairwell of the housing project in which the family lives. When she was interviewed, she was still showing the bruises and abrasions of the attack. The three youngest children, aged 18 months to 4 years, had chicken pox, and a 16-year-old daughter was at home, afraid to return to school because she was gang-raped last year and was terrified that this horrible event could happen again. She indicated that she wanted to finish school and become a cosmetologist. The 12-year-old daughter was nervous, shy, and withdrawn. Her father was currently incarcerated in another state, possibly to be released that year, and her mother was very definite that she never wanted to see him again. The 12-year-old daughter was the reason for the visit, because she was repeatedly running away from home and school, doing drugs, and meeting strangers (men) in bars and having unprotected sex with them. Her mother said, with tears pouring down her face, "This is how I started; is this how she is going to finish up?"

Over several visits, the children slowly opened up. The 12-year-old stated that she was angry with her mother for contracting HIV, that she knew her mother was going to die, and that she did not mind if she died as well. The 16-year-old said that another reason she didn't want to go to school was because she was afraid of returning home and finding her mother dead. There was no available transportation except when the older children, in their late teens and early 20s, came by. The apartment was clean and airy, and the older children were more than willing to help but were also busy with their own lives.

There were no male role models; grandma was sickly, with heart disease and diabetes, confined to a wheelchair, and living with her 35-year-old disabled daughter.

Support systems were extremely limited. This family was, to say the least, challenging, and really good outcomes will probably not be possible, but some things that were done were visits once a week to develop trust and explore resources within the family and the community of which they were unaware, such as door-to-door transportation for care, treatment, support groups, and the food and clothing bank; anonymous HIV testing for the other children, all of whom wanted to be tested (it was already known that the three youngest children were HIV+); regular medical assessment and intervention at a children-specific HIV center; and support groups at the children's center for the affected but not infected children.

The whole family willingly participated in some basic, easy-to-understand HIV and AIDS education at their home. Gradually they moved toward talking about dying and death and what this meant to the family. Over a period of months, the four oldest children decided that they would do their best to keep the family together by keeping the younger children when their mother died. This was discussed at a very nitty-gritty level, including financial needs, the probable illness of the younger children, the limitations that this would place on their lifestyles, and the commitment that would have to be made each and every day. It was profoundly moving to watch this family move into a very cohesive "we-are-all-in-this-together" structure.

The 12-year-old signed a written contract with the counselor agreeing that she would go to school regularly. *Regularly* meant starting with an agreed week, moving up to 2 weeks, and then a month. She is now attending full time, and although she sometimes expresses her intention of running away, she has not so far. She also has agreed within the contract that she will practice safer sex. However, as she has felt more secure she is leading a much healthier lifestyle. It is hoped that this will mean that her sexual activity can be replaced with more age-related activities.

The 16-year-old returned to school with the support of the school principal, the school counselor, and her teachers. The boys who had gang-raped her the previous year had dropped out of school, which took away a lot of her fears.

This family demonstrates the fact that even in really disastrous situations not only can something be salvaged, but there are always opportunities to enhance everyone's life, providing the family is willing to work together as a caring unit. The losses they face are not going to be easy for any of them, but because everyone is participating they should not have to cope with feelings of guilt, shame, or blame. They will survive and, one hopes, survive well. They now have a large network of community resources that are there for them, whatever the present holds or the future brings.

CONCLUSION

Worldwide, the number of women and children affected and infected by HIV continues to grow. In the United States, the spread is particularly evident in young women of color and women of Hispanic extraction of childbearing age.

The challenges are enormous, varied, and complex. There are no easy answers. Each client has a different history and needs. Effective intervention must attempt to meet these individual needs. Medical research, at long last and largely because of the spread of HIV, is addressing the specific issues of women and children. Safer sex is not nearly as easy as it sounds. Sex protection devices that a woman can control herself need to be developed. Children have practical and emotional needs that should be addressed before a parent's death. Health professionals need to feel comfortable in advocating pain management for kids and to be able to openly discuss feelings regarding dying and death.

There are no easy solutions. Being attentive, flexible, HIV-educated, and compassionate will help the climb up some of these seemingly insurmountable mountains.

REFERENCES

Bluebond-Langer, M. (1978). *The private worlds of dying children.* Princeton, NJ: Princeton University Press.

Cohn, B. (1993, August). Social security regulations: Women's symptoms finally recognized. *World, 28*, 6.

Denison, R. (1993, August). Can we put women in control? *World, 28*, 3.

de Selincourt, K. (1994, November). The family way. *Panos World Aids, 36*, 6–10.

Diaz, E. (1991, December/January). Public policy, women & HIV disease. *Siecus Report, 19*, 4–5.

Gilsenan, F. (ed.). (1994). *Reader's Digest legal problem solver.* Pleasantville, NY: The Reader's Digest Association.

Grubman, S., & Oleske, J. (1993). *The maturation of an epidemic: Update on pediatric HIV infection.* New Brunswick, NJ: University of Medicine and Dentistry of New Jersey, Department of Pediatrics.

Gutierrez, L. M. (1990). *Working with women of color: An empowerment perspective.* Washington, DC: National Association of Social Workers.

Hicks, J., & Hirsch, J. (1990, December). Young women and AIDS: A worldwide perspective. *Center for Population Options*, 1–2.

Holmes, S.A. (1994, April 29). Report sees rise in AIDS for children. *The New York Times*, p. A11.

Kellerman, V. (1994, August 24). Other end of the spectrum: AIDS strikes elderly. *The New York Times*, p. 14L1 10.

Lange, J. (1994). Zidovudine cuts mother-infant infections. *Global AIDS News, 1*, 10–11.

Levine, C., & Stein, G. L. (1994). *Orphans of the HIV epidemic.* New York: The Orphan Project.

National Community AIDS Partnership. (1992). *Voices of courage, a choir of needs.* Washington, DC: Author.

Osborn, J.E. (1991, April). Women in the trenches. *CDC HIV/AIDS Prevention Newsletter, 2*, 15.

Perez, E. (1991, December/January). Why women wait to be tested for HIV infection. *Siecus Report, 19*, 6–7.

Sack, F. (1992). *A romance to die for.* Deerfield Beach, FL: Health Communications, Inc.

U.S. Department of Health and Human Services. (1993). A guide to Social Security and SSI Disability benefits for people with HIV infection [Brochure]. Washington, DC: Author.

U.S. Department of Health and Human Services. (1994). Evaluation and management of early HIV infection (AHCPR Publication No. 94-0572). Rockville, MD: Author.

U.S. Public Health Service National Conference. (1991, August). Women and HIV infection. *Clinical Courier, 9*(6).

Wise, G. (1993). *A staff manual about AIDS and HIV infection for child care centers*. Immokalee, FL: Redlands Christian Migrant Association.

4

The Legal Issues:
Confusion, Clarification, Control

All have an interest in understanding legal issues that could have ramifications for those with HIV disease—for that could easily be any one of us.
—Allan Terl, *AIDS and the Law*

Not since the bubonic plague of 16th-century London has a disease caused such fear, hysteria, and myth among the world's population. In the early 1980s, when the retrovirus that appears to cause HIV/AIDS was first recognized, it was common to read newspaper headlines that described health professionals refusing to care for persons with AIDS, funeral directors geared up in outer space costumes before preparing for burial a person whose death was caused by AIDS, and individuals who were losing their jobs for no other reason than their bosses believed that they might be infected. Indeed, discrimination has frequently marked the societal and familial progression of the disease, often with dreadful consequences. Individuals have lost their livelihood, health insurance, and home and very survival ability because of attitudes that prevailed in the early years about those who were either infected or associated with those who were infected.

Families in this last decade of the 20th century have become more broadly interpreted. Levine (1994) suggests that there are certain essential characteristics that define family relationships. They are "permanence (at least in intention); commitment to mutuality of various forms of economic, social and emotional support; and a level of intimacy that distinguishes this bond from other less central attachments" (p. 5). Legally, same-sex marriages are not recognized in the United States, but "several communities have enacted laws extending spousal benefits to the partners of homosexual employees, including family-leave care for seriously ill homosexual partners. In a number of states homosexual couples have been allowed to adopt children" (Gilsenan, 1994, p. 284). Common law marriages are permitted in 14 states and even in these states must meet certain requirements. "Both of the people must be qualified to marry—that is they must be single, sane, competent, able to understand the meaning of the marital relationship, and in most states, of legal age to marry" (Gilsenan, 1994, p. 106). The two must live together and be seen as man and wife. While there is no formal written agreement to the marriage a legal divorce is needed to finish it. The counselor is wise to remember that nontraditional families receive little social support when it comes to laws, welfare systems, health care, insurance, and housing. Nevertheless, many of these non-traditional families "share deep, personal connections and are mutually entitled to receive and obligated to provide support of various kinds to the extent possible, especially in times of need" (Levine, 1994, p. 5).

AIDS is still usually a fatal disease. Preparing for the end of life is not some-thing that people do well legally. Older people may, but younger people see death as having little to do with them and rarely investigate or document their final wishes or their postdeath desires. When a disease becomes terminal, it becomes increasingly difficult to discuss such confrontational issues, with the result that thoughtful and directed decisions cannot be made. Not only does this heighten anxiety for infected and affected persons before death, but it frequently increases the emotional and financial cost to the survivors after death.

This chapter provides some guidelines for what can and should be done regard-ing a variety of legal issues. Do remember that states and nations have markedly different laws regarding almost everything and that legal issues and documents should always be discussed and drawn up with the input of a local attorney, a legal aid representative, or an HIV/AIDS-specific law group. Many regions within the United States now have such groups. They will usually be knowledgeable, helpful, and either free or very reasonable!

Confidentiality in HIV/AIDS takes on entirely new dimensions when the dis-closure of a positive status, however innocent, can have far-reaching consequences for the infected person, consequences that may begin immediately and continue throughout the course of the disease.

CONFIDENTIALITY

In the mid-1980s, Gary was an exemplary administrator in a large midwestern hospital. His life partner, Paul, was employed by the same institution. Gary was offered a disability insurance policy by his employer. To qualify he had to have what he was told were routine blood tests. The blood was drawn in the hospital emergency department. Five days later he was paged. It was Paul to tell him that the results of his blood test had already hit the gossip mill and that he was HIV-positive. Gary was devastated, enraged, and helpless to undo what had already thoughtlessly occurred, let alone come to terms with his new and unexpected posi-tive virus status.

Over the next 3 months, he was repeatedly warned that he was not doing his job well, after 15 years of superb evaluations. Realizing that the writing was on the wall and that his termination appeared to be imminent, he resigned. He and Paul moved to Florida where Paul died a few years ago from AIDS. Gary has only recently presented some signs and symptoms of disease process, but his former employer's lack of confidentiality and the effect that it had on both their lives has caused him to become an outspoken activist for the better understanding of AIDS care and treatment, particularly the emotional devastation that is so often part and parcel of this retrovirus.

State laws are written protecting the right to privacy of AIDS-infected individuals and their affected families, but they only work when we abide by them. Ignoring confidentiality may not only be illegal, but can provide the most horrifying acts of discrimination from which the involved party may never recover.

Always remember that confidential information is tied in some manner to some person or entity that can later be identified as related to that information. Anonymity, however, involves some manner of information without any identification that could later tie the information to the individual subject of it (Terl, 1992).

The issues surrounding confidentiality are most crucial at the time of testing. All testing should be informed, voluntary, and confidential. Clients should know how and where the testing information is stored and to whom the disclosure of a positive status will be made. Confidentiality is more challenging in settings such as foster care, residential facilities, schools, and detention institutions. The staff should receive ongoing education that stresses the emotional and physical harm and the legal consequences that can occur if there is a violation of the individual's right to privacy.

In Florida, disclosure of the test results is based on the need to know, which includes the test subject or his or her authorized representative, anyone legally authorized by the subject, health care providers or facilities for the purposes of diagnosis and treatment, employees of a health care facility who provide care and have a need to know, administrators and those who must practically be familiar with an employee's records, and a client's sexual and needle-sharing partners.

Need to know is defined as persons who provide patient care, or handle or process bodily fluids or tissue and have significant exposure. *Significant exposure* is defined as contact with the bodily fluids of clients, including through needle sticks and the worker (Crocket, 1993).

It is impossible to overemphasize the issues surrounding confidentiality and the importance of being knowledgeable regarding federal and state laws. That knowledge can make the difference between an empowered or a helpless client. Working or work-capable clients who believe that they may be experiencing employment-related discrimination are protected by the Americans with Disabilities Act (ADA).

THE AMERICANS WITH DISABILITIES ACT

The Americans with Disabilities Act became law on July 26, 1992. The ADA provides uniform, enforceable antidiscrimination protection inclusive of people with HIV disease. This is of particular importance in the area of employment as it specifically prohibits employers from discriminating against people with disabilities or people perceived to have disabilities, including people with HIV or AIDS. The ADA requires employers to make "reasonable accommodation" for workers with disabilities, including a flexible work schedule, restructuring of the job, time off for medical appointments, more flexible sick leave, or job reassignments and transfer (Pritchett, 1991). The ADA also prohibits employers from refusing to hire an applicant, from firing an employee, and from refusing to promote an employee because that person has HIV disease. Furthermore, employees cannot be routinely tested for HIV antibodies, nor can the test be included in a general physical examination as a condition of employment. The ADA as of July 1994 protects those organizations with 15 or more employees.

Unfortunately, the enactment of the law appears to lag behind the intent. According to the September/October 1994 issue of *Positively Aware* ("Chicago's Finest?" 1994), two potential police recruits were denied consideration for employment after testing positive for HIV in a required medical examination for employment by the Chicago Police Department. The American Civil Liberties Union is demanding that the police department be prohibited from testing recruits and that the applicants in question be allowed t\ continue to seek employment with the department. At the time of this writing, a decision has not yet been reached.

PREDEATH, DEATH, AND POSTDEATH WISHES

Some of the most challenging matters that need to be discussed and decided are those that surround predeath, death, and postdeath wishes. Bringing up financial and legal issues when there are visible signs of deteriorating health can seem and feel uncomfortable and tasteless. However, taking these steps will make a world of difference to the infected and affected. Before the death, it may mean the difference between absolute loss of personal control and empowerment, and after the death it may mean the survivor's ability to survive, physically, emotionally, and financially. There are a number of steps that can be chosen, and these include the appointment of a durable power of attorney for health care (also known as a health care agent or health care surrogate), convenience banking accounts, the writing of a living will and a will, and documentation implementing do-not-resuscitate (DNR) orders.

DURABLE POWER OF ATTORNEY

This is a legal document in which the client authorizes an individual, who is referred to as the agent, to act on his or her behalf in the event of the client's, referred to as the principal, incapacitation or incompetency. It ends only when and if the client has a guardian appointed, becomes competent again, or dies. The durable power of attorney may give the agent immediate authority to act on the principal's behalf or it may be designed to take effect at a specific time (Gilsenan, 1994).

The power of attorney can legally identify a broad range of tasks for the agent to perform that could include taking care of the principal's financial affairs, signing tax returns and insurance policies, selling real estate, buying and selling stocks and bonds, and making gifts with some restrictions. Usually the person who is dealing with the agent, also referred to as the attorney-in-fact, will ask to see a copy of the durable power of attorney to make sure the attorney-in-fact is acting within the scope of his or her authority. This offers some protection that the power will not be abused (Seiden, 1994).

DURABLE POWER OF ATTORNEY
FOR HEALTH CARE OR HEALTH CARE AGENT

This is another legal document that assigns an agent of the principal's choosing to clarify the principal's wishes regarding treatment and care only when the principal is no longer able to make those decisions. This may or may not be when the patient becomes terminal. It is often used in conjunction with a living will and authorizes the agent to make decisions consistent with the living will (Gilsenan, 1994). In the document, an alternate health care agent should be named in the event that the first agent is unable to perform this function, for whatever reason.

It cannot be emphasized enough how important it is to know whether your state allows the appointment of a health care agent (Alabama and Arkansas currently do not), whether your state allows your agent to refuse tube feeding, and how this must be documented to be implemented. It is crucial when choosing an agent and an alternate that these persons clearly understand the decisions that may have to be made and that they are comfortable taking on this responsibility and are willing to be the client's advocate if necessary. The agent ideally is knowledgeable, compassionate, understanding, responsible, and not easy to push around.

It helps if one's wishes and copies of the document are discussed and given to all family members so that a close relative who arrives on the scene as death approaches cannot change these wishes. Copies should be in the attorney's and doctor's offices, and with the medical chart if the client is in a medical institution. The document will require a different number of witnesses in different states, but one witness cannot be a spouse or blood relative.

A competent adult generally has the right to refuse medical treatment only when those wishes are expressed orally or in writing and he or she does not do so under duress (Gilsenan, 1994).

LIVING WILL

A living will is a signed, dated, and witnessed document that expresses those wishes regarding life-sustaining treatment should the person become incapable of taking responsibility for his or her own health care. The purpose of the living will is to protect individuals from the indignity and suffering of treatments that attempt to extend life inappropriately. A living will cannot be used to request euthanasia (Kaye, 1992).

Life-prolonging procedures that are addressed in the document usually include artificial sustenance and hydration, tube feeding, cardiac resuscitation, antibiotics, respiratory support, and surgery. A living will may also state if death is preferred in a facility or at home. The client can choose to have all or any one withheld or withdrawn at a time when rehabilitative measures are no longer effective. A living will provides direction for life partners, spouses, families, physi-

and attorneys when death becomes imminent. Physicians and hospitals are legally bound to honor valid living wills. The wording for a living will differs from state to state, but blank forms are frequently available in stationery stores and from Choice in Dying in New York. Remember to keep a living will separate from a regular will, which is usually opened only after death has occurred. Be sure to discuss its contents and whereabouts with one's nearest and dearest, physician, and attorney.

A living will only comes into effect when a diagnosis of a terminal stage is made by the physician and the patient can no longer communicate his or her wishes regarding life-prolonging treatment. In some states, a second medical opinion may be required. A living will may be revoked at any time, orally, in writing, by tearing up the document, or by writing *canceled* across it.

The intent of appointing a health care agent and writing a living will is to provide direction not only to one's immediate family but to physicians and health care facilities who now must support and comply with the individual's expressed wishes regarding his or her life and manner of death.

DO NOT RESUSCITATE

Although institutions are now obliged to honor their patients' wishes, it is important to remember that as more and more people are choosing to die at home surrounded by a familiar, comfortable, and comforting environment, the issue of DNR orders needs to be more comprehensively addressed. In the past, when a death of a terminally ill person occurred at home and the patient was not a hospice client, the emergency medical service (EMS) was called, and they would almost certainly commence resuscitation procedures. Very often the police would also arrive, and the home became a hive of inappropriate and escalating activity, frequently causing profound distress to the patient, caregivers, family, and friends. Do remember that in most states EMS technicians must attempt resuscitation even if the patient is terminally ill and has a living will ("Don't Leave Your Agent in the Dark," 1993).

Sometimes patients will need the services of EMS, for instance if they have fallen or wish to be taken to hospital for pain and symptom management; however, patients should receive only their own desired level of comfort care. The good news is that an increasing number of states are enacting laws that provide for prehospital or nonhospital DNR orders. Most states are required to develop a specific form, bracelet, or other symbol for patients to carry on their person (More About Nonhospital DNR Orders," 1993). In Florida, for example, the prehospital or nonhospital DNR form was developed by the Department of Health and Rehabilitative Services. It must be completed and signed by the attending physician, the patient or health care agent or guardian, and two witnesses. It is a good idea to keep it in a visible place so that it is readily available if EMS is called. The refrigerator door is an ideal location as anyone can find the refrigerator door no matter how panicked and anxious they may feel.

Making plans is important, but frequently people are handicapped because they do not know where to find papers, telephone numbers, keys, and so forth. The following form is designed to help and should be placed where it can readily be seen. A friend keeps hers under the glass of her desktop in her home study.

Whereabouts of Documents

The following important documents, names, telephone numbers, keys, bank accounts, and so forth may be found as listed below:

KEY: *(Write in locations on the lines.)*
A. *Attorney—telephone no.:* _____
P. *Physician—telephone no.:* _____
M. *Minister—telephone no.:* _____
B. *Bank(s)—telephone no(s).:* _____
S. *Safe deposit box—address:* _____
H. *Home—location:* _____
W. *Work—location:* _____
Living will: _____
Disposition of organs and/or body: _____
Will: _____
Spouse's death certificate: _____
Marriage license: _____
Safe deposit box key and who is authorized to sign: _____

Life insurance policies: _____
Accident and health policies: _____
Charge card benefits: _____
Social Security Card or number: _____
Passport or number: _____
Bank books: _____
Loans: _____
Property mortgage and/or lease: _____
Deed to home: _____
Title to car, motorcycle, boat, and so forth: _____
Income tax return, receipts, and canceled checks: _____
Certificate of ownership of cemetery lot: _____
Property damage and flood insurance policies: _____
If naturalized, citizenship papers: _____
Military discharge papers: _____
Jewelry: _____
Other important documents or valuables: _____

As more heterosexual women and children become infected, the issues of child custody and guardianship arise not only for an orphaned sick child but for an uninfected child. Addressing these issues is usually extraordinarily stressful but is better done sooner rather than later. Do remember that the parents may be legal or illegal immigrants and may neither have relatives in this country nor want their immigrant status known for fear of detention and subsequent deportation.

CUSTODY AND GUARDIANSHIP DECISIONS

Parents are normally responsible for the care and nurturing of their children. When circumstances prevent one or both parents from fulfilling this obligation, courts determine who shall have custody of the child. The state's interest is in seeing that the child is protected, as much as possible, from the harmful effects of divorce, separation, or death.

Parents can, before death, make guardianship arrangements with a consenting relative. However, as many of these children come from poor, minority families, placement may be more challenging because the intended caregiver could have the same social and economic problems as the natural mother. If a parent fails to make a written declaration indicating his or her preference of a guardian, the court is directed to give preference to a person who is related by blood or marriage to the ward. This may or may not match the parents' desires, which reinforces the need to make informed decisions early.

Anyone who provides substantial services to the child in a professional or business capacity may not be allowed to provide guardianship. If parents are designating a person to be appointed as guardian after their death, it must be in writing. This is known as testamentary guardianship. It can assign custody rights and the management of the child's property, or there can be a guardian for each task.

Before making a testamentary guardianship, do make certain that the chosen person is willing to take on this enormous and lasting responsibility; one or two alternatives are named in the event that the first person becomes unable to care for the children; and the chosen individual understands the beliefs, customs, values, and religious practices of the biological family.

Difficulties may also arise because of divorce, separation, or death when the other parent is lesbian, gay, or has AIDS. Courts may not grant custodial rights to that biological parent although there does appear to be a trend toward more acceptance of nontraditional relationships.

Choosing a guardian is a thoughtful process with far-reaching consequences. Children deserve the very best that can be done, but it also has to be recognized that choices may be very limited, and an optimum situation may not be possible. Writing a will can help to identify and legalize the needs of all family members. A written will can make the difference between survival and financial disaster, recovery and ruin for the survivor.

WILLS

Homosexual men and women, and people living together who are not married, have a special need to have a will. The law makes no provisions for lovers, friends, or any other person not related by blood or marriage to the person who died (Martelli, Peltz, & Messina, 1987). Wills provide for the surviving partner, regardless of the legal status of the relationship. Unfortunately, people frequently find discussing wills uncomfortable, unromantic, and a reminder that life is finite. They will put off any conversation or documentation until death occurs, when, of course, it is much too late. When death occurs without a will, the state will distribute the property according to the state's laws of inheritance and distribution that identify who gets what. The law generally believes that we would rather leave our property to our immediate family, which may or may not be true! This could mean that our nearest and dearest such as a life partner may not see a penny.

A last will and testament stipulates how assets are to be distributed, identifies an executor to oversee the estate, and names a guardian for minors and a beneficiary for the residuary estate. The residuary estate is the property that remains after all bequests, taxes, and expenses have been met. Wills are not expensive, complicated, or time consuming. Will forms can be bought at many stationers, but it is wiser to have a will drawn up by an attorney who can provide advice regarding state laws and any complicating factors. If this is too expensive, contact the local AIDS community programs and ask them where you can seek legal help.

CONVENIENCE ACCOUNTS

This is a banking account that is only for those who have an absolutely trustworthy person as the signatory. The signatory can sign checks in the event of the principal's physical incapacity and hospitalization. If there is mental incompetence, the signatory can handle the checkbook. This can be an enormous assistance and an enormous temptation, so be extremely cautious before choosing a signatory.

COHABITATION

This is usually defined as living together without marrying. It is not a common-law marriage and provides little legal protection for either partner. No state recognizes a homosexual marriage, although some cities, counties, and states allow unmarried couples to register as domestic partners. Unless there is a will or some kind of "living-together" agreement, entitlements to assets will only be those held in each individual's name.

Joint property agreements, legally documented, ensure the fair distribution of goods and real estate. If no will is made but there is a joint property agreement, the assigned assets will go to the survivor.

CONCLUSION

It's a good idea to review all legal documents with an attorney every 2–3 years as laws can be altered. Wills should comply with the state in which one is living. Wills written in other states should be reviewed and revised to conform with the present state of residence.

This chapter has addressed some of the legal issues that are important to each and every one of us. Making our legal lives current can make a profound difference to the way that we will be treated in a terminal stage. Our families, whomever they may be, will be guided and grateful for the postdeath plans that are made.

In this technological age, it has become increasingly easy to make thoughtful, informed, and legally binding arrangements as attorneys now have instant access to computerized blank forms that may be filled out to conform with your clients' wishes and state law.

Taking care of legal issues is best accomplished when the shadows of illness are not on us, but when we are in good health and have a clear mind and emotions will not have such a confusing impact on decision making. Resolving legal issues provides peace of mind, tranquility, and long-range results that cannot be overemphasized.

REFERENCES

Chicago's Finest? (1994, September/October). *Positively Aware*, p. 5.

Crocket, P. H. (Ed.). *AIDS and the law*. Miami Beach, FL: Crocket & Franklin.

Don't leave your agent in the dark. (1993, Winter). *Choice in Dying News, 4*, 1–6.

Gilsenan, F. (1994). *Reader's Digest legal problem solver*. Pleasantville, NY: Reader's Digest Association.

Kaye, P. (1992). *Symptom control in palliative care*. Essex, CT: Hospice Education Institute.

Levine, C. (1994). AIDS and the changing concept of family. In R. Bor & J. Elford (Eds.), *The family & HIV* (pp. 3–22). Trowbridge, Wiltshire, England: Redwood Books.

Martelli, J. L., Peltz, F. D., & Messina, W. (1987). *When someone you know has AIDS: A practical guide*. New York: Crown.

More about nonhospital DNR orders. (1993, Summer). *Choice in Dying News, 2*, 3.

Pritchett, J. (Ed.). (1991). *The HIV/AIDS book: Information for workers* (4th ed.). Washington, DC: Occupational Health & Safety Department, Service Employees International Union.

Seiden, L. S. (1994, October 24). Make a plan in case you become disabled. *The Sun Sentinel Business Weekly*, p. 28.

Terl, A. H. (1992). *AIDS and the law*. Washington, DC: Hemisphere.

5

Untangling the Bureaucratic Maze

Money speaks sense in a language all nations understand. —Aphra Behn (1640–1689)

Of all diseases known to us, HIV/AIDS is surely the one that has had the most profound financial impact on nations, regions, states, counties, families, and individuals. AIDS has reached all corners of our world, and its economic cost continues to escalate.

Health care reform is on the political agenda of many comparatively wealthy countries as maintaining their citizens' well-being takes ever larger chunks out of their gross national products. Add the cost of HIV/AIDS to the health budget, and the picture becomes even gloomier.

According to Kenneth South (1993), the cost of treating an individual adult with AIDS in the United States from the time of diagnosis of HIV infection until the time of death has dropped from a high of $147,000 in 1987 to a cost of $32,000 in 1992. The lower cost of treatment has occurred for a variety of reasons including better use of less costly medications, better medical intervention that generally results in the individual spending far less time in intensive care units and acute care hospitals, and a focus on managed care and increased financial support to keep the individual in the comfort and reassurance of their own home. However, although the costs of caring are dropping, nothing can alter the fact that the people who are most affected are those between the ages of 20–49, in the prime of their lives at a time when they are economically productive, taxpayers, childbearers, and the mainstays of national economies.

In Africa, Latin America, and Asia where HIV is spread mainly through heterosexual intercourse, it is having a socioeconomic impact out of all proportion to the people infected. Virtually every person who dies from an AIDS-related opportunistic infection leaves dependent family members who may be totally impoverished because of the costs in time and money of caring for and burying him or her. In Thailand, the health care costs alone for a person with AIDS are estimated to be one third to one half of the average annual family income. Over the next 6 years, developing countries will spend close to $1 billion on health care for AIDS patients (Merson, 1994).

Indirect costs include the loss of employees; the inability to till lands, grow crops, and raise livestock; orphaned children; increasing training and labor costs; and decreasing personal income. Even building ties with wealthier nations may prove to be a "Catch-22" situation. According to Mexican AIDS activist Juan Chavez (1994), as Mexico promotes an image of self-sufficiency, needy AIDS organizations find it increasingly difficult to receive international funds to fight HIV. "Remember, we are members of NAFTA now," said Chavez (1994, p. 24). This is happening not only in Mexico, but in other countries such as Chile and Malaysia.

Within the continental and contiguous United States, there are a variety of financial aid programs that can benefit and support individuals infected with HIV. This chapter presents some of them, but do research the accessibility and availability of programs in your own area so that you can provide your clients with accurate and current information. Knowledge is power, and this helps the individual to develop and maintain a sense of support and control. There are few things more frightening in a capitalistic society than fearing that you may lose all your financial assets. Health professionals have a wonderful opportunity to assist their working clients by encouraging them to stay employed for as long as possible. Work reflects clients' belief in themselves and enables them to stay independent.

EMPLOYMENT AND HIV/AIDS

Jobs usually carry benefits, and one of the most important is the employer's health insurance benefit. An HIV-positive (HIV+) status may mean, as with any other chronic illness, that a change in job will cause the loss of health insurance as a new insurance company will almost certainly exclude the individual, citing the HIV status as a preexisting condition.

Another benefit of keeping a job is a salary, thus enabling the individual to meet basic survival needs. However, jobs also go a long way toward enhancing self-esteem, providing social contact, and developing support systems. So it is important to know whether a client's place of employment has a catastrophic illness policy, how it is implemented, and what the content is. If there isn't one, now is the time to encourage employers to develop one.

The Service Employees International Union in its HIV/AIDS book *Information for Workers* (Pritchett, 1991) has suggested the following guidelines for AIDS and other catastrophic illnesses.

Catastrophic Illness Policy

1. Workers with catastrophic illnesses should be able to continue working as long as they are physically able to perform the job.
2. Employers should attempt to provide reasonable accommodation for workers with catastrophic illnesses. Job modifications might include flextime, job sharing, more breaks, and working from home if the worker wishes.

3. Confidentiality of workers with long-term illnesses should be maintained, allowing them to determine who should have information about their diagnosis.
4. HIV antibody or antigen testing as a condition of employment should be prohibited.
5. Employers should provide HIV/AIDS education to all employees, including supervisory and management personnel. This should be a cooperative program developed between the union and management.
6. Employee benefit plans should be adjusted to accommodate the needs of people with catastrophic illnesses. Features might include granting sick leave to attend medical appointments, granting short-term disability leave for hospitalization or recuperation, granting long-term disability to those who need an extended medical leave, and ensuring that plans cover home care, hospice care, extended care, and necessary prescription drugs.
7. Workers with catastrophic illnesses should be treated with compassion and understanding.

Discrimination

If there is any apparent or real act of discrimination in the workplace, the client should immediately seek legal council from an attorney who is familiar with state laws and HIV issues. These attorneys can be found by contacting local HIV/AIDS community services or by calling LAMBDA Legal Defense and Education Fund in New York City.

Health insurance has become an increasing concern to those who are unemployed with preexisting conditions and those who are employed but because of ill health may not feel capable of working each and all day. It behooves the counselor to become knowledgeable regarding the convoluted minefield of health insurance and to be aware of the available options.

Private Health Insurance

Private health insurance in the United States is undergoing many changes that one hopes will help to make the insured's health life easier. Insurance premium costs in 1994 seem to have stabilized, more policies are portable, and there are more options for small organizations, the self-employed, and younger retirees. Generally, health insurance companies cover basic medical care, hospitalization, and catastrophic health care.

Basic medical coverage. This covers the physician's fees for either an office visit or the hospital outpatient department, laboratory and radiology services, and sometimes prescription drugs. Charges reflect the customary charge in a given area. In Ft. Lauderdale, for instance, the usual price for fixing a broken toe may be $400, and where the physician charges more than this, the insured is expected to pay the difference.

Copayment or coinsurance. Most insurance companies have an established copayment of either 10 or 20% that is paid by the insured at the time services are rendered.

Hospitalization coverage. Most health insurance companies pay all or part of a hospital stay in a semiprivate room, which is defined as a room shared by two people. There is usually a maximum dollar amount per year that the insured will have as a copayment. Other services that are usually covered are the primary care physician, specialist, and surgeon; operation and recovery room, intensive care, and other special units; medication, drugs, intravenous therapy, and solutions; anesthesia and oxygen services; inhalation and respiratory therapy; laboratory, x-ray, and other diagnostic procedures; prescribed special diets; and short-term physical therapy.

Major medical or catastrophic health coverage. This covers the cost of serious or prolonged illnesses, expensive surgery, or other expensive treatments. Services that should be covered are prolonged hospitalization, skilled nursing facility, hospice, and home health care. There is usually an annual deductible and a 20–30% copayment by the insured.

Group insurance. The majority of working people receive health insurance through their employer, union, or professional organization. Group policy premiums are generally lower than individual policies. Some employers pay the full premium, but as costs have escalated individuals are more frequently expected to contribute and have the contribution deducted from their paychecks. Many group policies can be extended to include family members. A big advantage of group coverage is that an individual cannot be dropped from the policy.

If the insured is self-covered, it is important to remind the client to pay the premium. Insurance companies may or may not have a grace period, meaning that coverage continues after the date for payment of the next premium. If the client misses the grace period deadline, all coverage is dropped.

Health Maintenance Organizations (HMOs)

HMOs have not always had the best publicity, but they are growing concerns and have a lot to offer at a lower monthly premium if staying with one's own physician is not important. An HMO has a list of physicians, and the client chooses a primary care physician from that list. The primary care physician is then responsible for the delivery of health care and will make referrals for specialized care if it is needed. Some of the advantages of joining an HMO are that the monthly premium covers the majority of costs; there is unlimited access to health care services; clients do not have to file claim forms; and, if it is a well-run HMO, there is access to health care 24 hours a day, 7 days a week. The disadvantages of an HMO are that choices are limited regarding specialists; unless the client wishes to pay privately, outside opinions and treatment cannot be sought; basic treatments may not be administered by a physician; and fewer tests and services may be offered.

Preferred Provider Organization (PPOs)

PPOs are organizations in which physicians have agreed to be paid lower fees for services in return for becoming a provider for an insurer. By doing this, employers and insurers control health care costs. The insured can go to any physician on the PPO list at any time, and as PPOs become more popular with physicians, these lists are becoming larger. Visiting a non-PPO physician will usually mean that the client will pay more or have the claim rejected. There may be a preauthorization clause that requires the primary care physician to notify the hospital or specialist before the delivery of these services.

It cannot be emphasized enough how important it is to remind clients to read insurance policies several times very carefully, particularly the exceptions and the amount of lifetime coverage, which are usually listed at the end of the policy. Before signing up, the client should ask every question that does not appear to be addressed in the policy and not put a signature to paper or pen to check until there is a feeling of understanding and trust.

Rejection of a Claim

This can be extremely aggravating and may be completely reasonable!

There are several steps to take: If there is an agent, tell the client to call him or her and see if he or she will be willing to speak with the insurer; call the claims department and request a written reason for the denial and documentation of the policy terms that allows the company to deny it; follow up the call with a written protest detailing the occurrence; keep copies, documentation dates, and names of the people who receive letters and telephone calls. The denial may be because papers were filled out incorrectly or more details are needed from the physician, so the client should not give up too easily.

If no satisfaction occurs, have the client contact the state's department of insurance, many of whom have regional offices. If they believe the claim is reasonable, they may intervene. If all else fails, it may be necessary to hire an attorney and take the matter to court.

Being persistent is probably the most powerful weapon—daily phone calls do not have to be angry or hostile, but making them reminds the insurer that the client expects a positive outcome.

Jobs and Health Insurance

Today, it is a norm for life, health, or disability insurers to screen all potential clients for HIV disease. If the test is returned as HIV+, it is almost certain that coverage will be denied with, according to Richard Greenberg (1994), one major exception, the government at all levels: federal, state, county, and city. "As employers with large work forces, government entities provide all of their employees with group insurance coverage with guaranteed access for all, regardless of HIV status" (Greenberg, 1994, p. 5). Government programs will offer a variety of choices and will pay the major portion of the monthly premiums. Greenberg went on to say that "with a government job and just a little pre-planning on your part, you can get yourself well insured for any eventuality, as I did" (p. 5).

In Florida, government bodies offer a veritable cornucopia of insurance options, including joining a PPO or an HMO, which include a prescription drug plan with a small copayment for each prescription, supplemental hospitalization insurance, low-cost group life insurance, dental plans, and accident and disability plans. The beauty of these plans is that HIV+ individuals are not excluded, the costs are low, and some policies pay cash for being in the hospital that can be used in any way that the employee wishes. Although government salaries are notoriously low, the benefits are incredibly worthwhile.

Being knowledgeable and organized when job hunting can have remarkable results, and again can make the difference between living well and merely existing.

The Consolidated Omnibus Budget Reconciliation Act

In 1985, a law called the Consolidated Omnibus Budget Reconciliation Act (COBRA) was passed that entitled employees leaving their jobs continued health coverage from 18 months to a maximum of 36 months. Companies with 20 or more employees must offer this coverage to an employee when employment ends under the following circumstances: termination from employment, a cutback in work hours causing loss of entitlement to benefits, whenever a worker becomes entitled to Medicare, and whenever a worker's dependent child reaches the age when he or she is no longer eligible for coverage under the employer's health plan (Pritchett, 1991). Employees who are fired for gross misconduct are ineligible for the continuance of this coverage.

COBRA has proven remarkably helpful to a lot of people, but it can still be very costly as the individual now has to pay the entire monthly premium plus a small administration fee. Something else to remember is that if a major medical problem develops during the continuation of the coverage, getting other health insurance at a later time may prove difficult. Nevertheless, COBRA provides a safety net and a sense of security at a time when other coverage may be difficult to find immediately.

LIFE INSURANCE POLICIES

Life Insurance

Policies are written for a specified beneficiary to receive a specified amount of compensation when the policyholder dies. There are three parties to life insurance coverage: the insured, on whose death the insurance company pays out the benefits of the policy; the insurer, the insurance company itself; and the beneficiary, to whom benefits are paid on the death of the insured (Terl, 1992).

Viatical Settlement Companies

A relatively new business has developed, life insurance buyouts. A buyout means that a viatical settlement company (*viatical* comes from the Latin for "money given to a traveler") purchases the life insurance policies of people who are terminally ill. It provides an opportunity for the insured to have cash on hand and therefore to relieve some of the financial distress that all too frequently accompanies a life-limiting illness, particularly in the United States. It also can mean not only that everyday living is improved, but that home foreclosure may be averted, repossession of household goods stopped, some dreams can be accomplished, and financial independence achieved. It pays a price lower than the face value of the life insurance policy to the insured for an irrevocable assignment of the right to the benefits on the death of the insured.

Taking this step requires care, thought, and caution. Viatical settlement companies are covered by few federal or state laws because they only recently came into being. They are in the business to make money at a time when clients are at their most vulnerable and when the company can anticipate that little more than 1 or 2 years will pass before it enjoys a return of its original investment plus an excellent profit—not a bad deal! Companies offer to buy the policy for anywhere from 35 to 85% of its face value, and some companies do not state what percentage they will pay, so be very certain to tell the client to ask.

The criteria for buying varies and may include some of the following: a life expectancy of 48 months or less; T cell counts below 320; medical records are authorized to be released; the policy was in force at least 2 years before diagnosis; any bankruptcy proceedings are disclosed; and whether any public assistance is being received.

The applicant's physician must provide documentation of a terminal illness. Each beneficiary of the policy must confirm in writing that he or she understands the reason for the transaction and that he or she waives claim to the proceeds. Dependent children under the age of 18 are to be sufficiently provided for, either from the proceeds of the sale or by other means. The percentage that is paid is based on the client's medical condition. A higher rate is paid for a shorter life prognosis.

The Process

A questionnaire and release forms are sent to the insured after the insured has contacted a viatical settlement company. When the application is returned to the company, they will send authorization forms to the applicant's physician and the life insurance company so that their records are made available for review. Some companies act as brokers and put the insurance policy up for outside bids; others are independently financed and payment will be instant on approval of the purchase by the company.

Buyer Beware

Before taking this major step, it is extremely important that the client seek advice from independent legal, financial, and income tax professionals. Questions your client should ask include the following:

1. What is the company's average payment turnaround time?
2. Is everything strictly confidential?
3. How long has the company been in business?
4. Is the settlement money kept in an escrow account until the transaction is complete?
5. Is the company user friendly?
6. Will this affect benefits being received from other programs such as Social Security and Medicare?
7. Is this considered taxable income?

Other Alternatives

There may be other options that do not require selling the life insurance policy but will provide money when it is most needed. For instance, check with the insurance carrier to find out whether an accelerated program is offered. If there is, the client may be eligible to borrow funds against the life insurance, often at a very low interest rate. It may be possible to cash in the policy and obtain the policy's cash surrender value.

If a buyout seems a good idea, the client should shop around and make the best deal possible. Arlene Terry, a person with AIDS (PWA) whose greatest wish was to keep her home, sought the services of a viatical settlement company and said "critics who call the practice morbid ought to walk a day in my shoes. . . . My pride and dignity and ability to make choices in life are way more important than these people and their morality issues" (Turnbull, 1992, p. A1).

For those people with HIV who have exhausted their personal resources, Social Security can provide a lifeline of support. That lifeline comes in the form of monthly Social Security disability benefits and Supplemental Security Income (SSI) payments, Medicare and Medicaid coverage, and a variety of services available to people who receive disability benefits from Social Security (U.S. Department of Health & Human Services, 1993).

SOCIAL SECURITY BENEFITS

Many people who are HIV-infected are receiving some form of federal and state financial aid. However, every avenue of assistance should be explored to see if any form of compensation is available. In its most basic form, the Social Security Administration's task is to give out money to eligible clients. It does not give sympathy or advice but does provide a lot of information and practical economic support.

Social Security Disability Benefits (SSDI)

SSDI, as discussed earlier in this book (see chapter 3), provides a monthly cash payment to those people who have paid Social Security taxes and have earned work credits toward eventual benefits. The number of work credits that are needed to qualify for disability benefits depends on the age of the individual at the time of the disability. The maximum number of credits that can be earned each year is 4. Nobody needs more than 40 credits to qualify, and younger people may be able to qualify with as few as 6. Widows and widowers aged 50 years and older could be eligible through the Social Security record of a deceased spouse. Disabled children aged 18 or older could be eligible for a dependents' benefits on the Social Security record of a parent who is receiving retirement or disability benefits or on the record of a parent who has died. Children under the age of 18 qualify for dependents' benefits on the record of a parent who is receiving retirement or disability benefits or on the record of a parent who has died.

Benefits are based on the person's income throughout his or her work life, meaning that a higher income generally means a higher benefit. It is a good idea to verify that Social Security has an accurate record of all work earnings. If the amount is incorrect, the local Social Security Administration office should be contacted immediately, proof should be given of actual wages earned, and a correction can then be made.

In each state, there is an agency usually identified as the Disability Determination Service that evaluates disability claims. The Disability Determination Service addresses the following:

- the severity of the impairment and how much it interferes with the ability to work from the perspective of daily activities, social functioning, and the ability to complete tasks in a timely manner.
- whether the impairment is on the list of impairments that for HIV-related conditions is quite lengthy and has additional criteria for HIV-infected women.

Remember to tell the client that

- There is no income test from sources other than work.
- There are no questions referring to assets.
- After 2 years on disability, qualification occurs for Medicare.

The client can start the process by contacting a local HIV/AIDS case management program, a social worker attached to a medical institution, or the local Social Security Administration office.

The Social Security Administration will need the following:

- Social Security number
- birth certificate
- Social Security numbers and birth certificates for family members signing up on the client's record
- the most recent W-2 form (or tax return if self-employed)

The Social Security Administration has stated that it "is committed to helping all men, women and children with HIV infection learn more about the disability programs [they] administer. And if you qualify for benefits, [they] are just as committed to ensuring that you receive them as soon as possible" (U.S. Department of Health and Human Services, 1993, p. 4). Clients should be very involved in helping the process along by

- personally documenting the signs and symptoms of the illness from its earliest stages and updating the documentation regularly; a health diary keeps dates and times comprehensively.
- reminding health care professionals to carefully document the course of the illness.
- documenting if, when, and why a job was lost through ill health.
- giving Social Security detailed health records when applying for disability.

Too much documentation is infinitely better than too little!

If the application is turned down, encourage your client to be persistent and follow up repeatedly on the original claim, refile, plead the case, or, if there appears to be a good case and all else fails, sue.

Supplemental Security Income

SSI is a program that pays monthly benefits to people with low incomes and limited assets who are 65 or older, blind, or disabled. It is funded through the federal government's general revenues and is for those who have either never paid Social Security taxes or whose income falls below the federal government's poverty level. The benefits available from SSI will differ from state to state as they are dependent on the level of the state's contribution. The local Social Security Administration office will be able to provide the client with benefits information. Criteria for receiving SSI include the following:

* limited assets, which generally for individuals are under $2,000 or for couples under $3,000. Items such as one home, a car valued under $4,500, and most personal belongings are not included in measuring personal income. Food stamps, food, clothing, or housing received through a nonprofit organization or government-sponsored programs are also not counted.
* residence within the United States or Northern Mariana Islands.
* having U.S. citizenship, or being a legally admitted alien or an alien living within the United States who is in the process of applying for residency status. (Note: At the time of this writing, entitlements for all aliens are currently under congressional review and may change.)
* having an income that falls below the federal government's poverty-level index.

To qualify, the client should contact the local Social Security Administration office.

Medicare

Medicare is a major government-run health insurance program that helps to pay for health care for people over 65 years of age regardless of their income or assets, and for certain people under the age of 65. Medicare coverage is generally earned by those whose jobs are covered by Social Security, or by a railroad or the federal government. People who qualify for Medicare under the age of 65 are recipients of SSDI, persons suffering from kidney failure who need dialysis or a kidney transplant, or both. Medicare is divided into Part A and Part B.

Part A. Part A pays for hospitalization, inpatient care in a skilled nursing facility, posthospital home health care, or hospice care. There are deductibles for hospitalization and nursing home care.

Part B. Part B helps to pay for doctors' services, outpatient services, and other services not covered by Part A.

Deductibles. Both programs have some form of deductible. For more detailed information regarding Medicare, have the client contact the local Social Security Administration office.

Medicaid

Medicaid is the other major government-run health insurance policy. Medicaid is generally available to people with low incomes and those who qualify for SSI. Medicaid is funded jointly by federal and state governments and is required to cover certain services, including inpatient and outpatient hospital care and physician services. Individual states will cover other services, and each state formulates its own regulations on eligibility, coverage, and benefits. Have the client call the local Medicaid office for detailed information. Again, if a client's application is turned down the first time, he or she should keep on trying. Eligibility criteria change, as do individuals' financial, physical, and mental states. Persistence can truly pay! Individual states may also have a separate Medicaid waiver program specifically designed for PWAs that provides comprehensive and broad coverage through a case-managed program.

CASE MANAGEMENT

Case management refers to the process of evaluating clients' service needs, planning and arranging service delivery, and monitoring both client progress and provider compliance with the plan of care. Case managers develop and reassess the plan of care and coordinate formal and informal service delivery systems (Florida Department of Health and Human Services, 1992). In other words, an individual case manager is appointed who may be a registered nurse, a social worker, or another health professional. The case manager is then assigned a specified number of clients, with a specific amount of money provided for each client on an annual basis. The case manager contracts with other providers to provide the medical, emotional, and physical support systems that are needed for the client's well-being. When case management is interpreted and delivered with compassion and efficiency, it provides a cost-contained, timely, and positive intervention that is keyed to the client's individual needs. The results are heartwarming and effective.

FOOD STAMPS

Food stamps offer lower income people stamps issued by the government to pay for food items at authorized grocery stores. Most grocery stores seem to be authorized. Stamps cannot be used to buy alcohol, tobacco, pet food, cleaning products, medicine, ready-to-eat foods, or vitamins. Although this is a federal program, it is administered by state social service or welfare departments and, once again, the income and assets limits will vary according to the eligibility criteria for each state.

To apply for food stamps, the intended recipient must usually apply in person or, if this is not possible, another person can be appointed to appear instead. If the application is accepted, the recipient will receive an Authorization to Participate that must be exchanged each month at the food stamp office to receive more stamps. Guidelines for eligibility differ by individual state. Requirements include proof of residence for everyone living in the household; photo identification; birth certificate of each household member; proof of citizenship; and information regarding income, insurance, and current bills. There are also requirements for mail delivery of food stamps. The many requirements may sound extraordinary, but food stamps can be acquired. Perseverance is the name of the game.

SPECIFIC FEDERAL PROGRAMS

Each state has a federal grant program that helps to pay for some HIV medications for people who need assistance, but who don't have private insurance or have only partial private insurance and who meet certain financial and medical requirements. These programs were designed mainly to help people who need financial help, but don't qualify for Medicaid. The requirements for the federal program vary from state to state. The local DSS office or the AIDS Information Office of the state health department can explain how the federal grant programs work. The state health department can provide information regarding its HIV Drug Assistance program.

AID TO FAMILIES WITH DEPENDENT CHILDREN

Aid to Families with Dependent Children (AFDC) is a federal government welfare program that supplies the funding money and basic guidelines for a program that helps "provide children and their families with the basic necessities of life while also trying to ensure that the families it supports stay together" (Gilsenan, 1994, p. 24).

In some areas of the United States, HIV/AIDS is spreading most rapidly among women of childbearing age, adolescents, and young children. HIV/AIDS is a family disease. AFDC may be the financial intervention that helps to maintain the integrity of the family unit at a time when it would otherwise splinter apart.

AFDC is administered at state and local levels and again is individually interpreted in each state. The state also decides the amount of money that the applicant will receive. Eligibility is determined by the needs of the child or children in each family. Areas that are addressed for qualification are levels of deprivation, age, relationships, and economic support.

Deprivation

Deprivation addresses the lack of support from one or both parents because of prolonged absence from the home, parental physical or mental disability, death of one or both parents, or unemployment.

Age

The child must be under 18 and unmarried.

Relationship

The applicant must be a parent or relative of the child.

Income

The local AFDC office compares the family's financial resources to the amount that the state has decided a family that size requires in order to live. There is a determination of the family's net assets, including the net value of property other than one's own home, certain vehicles, bank accounts, bonds, and some life insurance policies. The local office weighs the net assets and any other pertinent criteria against the state's payment formula. This determines the amount of the benefit that will be paid.

Applicants are expected to reveal the whereabouts of an absent parent if this is known. They may be required to participate in a job-training or job-seeking program as the hope of AFDC is that families can become self-supporting.

FAMILY AND MEDICAL LEAVE ACT

In 1993, President Clinton signed into federal law the Family and Medical Leave Act (FMLA). The law applies to employers who have more than 50 employees. It provides up to 12 weeks of unpaid leave annually for those who have worked for the company at least 1 year or who work more than 1,250 hours or more a year (25 hours per week) and whose salaries are not in the top 10% of that particular company.

Leave is given specifically for the employee's own serious illness; for that of a very ill spouse, minor child, minor adopted child, parent, newborn, or foster child within a year of that child's arrival; and for an adult child if incapable of self-care. Excluded are nonmarried partners, in-laws, siblings, grandchildren, and grandparents.

Employees must usually give 30 days notice and should be prepared to verify the need with a health care provider's certification. The law also requires that employees be reinstated to their former jobs or to similar duties, although layoffs are permitted. If health insurance premiums are paid by the employer, the employer must continue to do so during the employee's absence.The leave does not have to be taken in one lump but can be taken in short increments, such as a morning a week.

The FMLA can obviously be of great assistance to those infected with HIV where sudden and serious illness can often be followed by good health over a period of years.

COMMUNITY-BASED HIV/AIDS ORGANIZATIONS

An enormous number of local agencies are now supplying a multitude of services. In many cities and rural areas, there is the opportunity to access a variety of resources that include HIV/AIDS support groups for gays, lesbians, heterosexuals, women, children, chemical dependents, and long-term survivors; educational programs that provide information regarding research, clinical trials, legal issues, Social Security, stress management, and sexually transmitted diseases; practical programs that provide free food and clothing banks, meals delivered to the home, pet care, transportation (always a huge need), preschool day care, adult day care, residential facilities, independent living facilities, and legal aid.

CONCLUSION

Confronting the bureaucratic maze appears overwhelmingly confusing and impossible, particularly if one is sick. Health professionals and friends can be invaluable when they learn the systems, make phone calls, see that documentation is intact, and accompany clients to interviews. Encouraging clients to take one step at a time and to be persistent and patient and refuse to be deterred can provide long-term rewards that can significantly affect the physical and emotional effects caused by this retrovirus called HIV.

Most of all, do not allow the client to feel embarrassed or too proud to take advantage of government assistance. The programs and the money are there to help. They should be fully used in good conscience!

REFERENCES

Chavez, C. (1994, September/October). Prevention still the best vaccine. *Positively Aware, 24.*

Florida Department of Health and Human Services. (1992). *Description of services under the waiver.* Tallahassee, FL: Author.

Gilsenan, F. (1994). *Readers Digest legal problem solver.* Pleasantville, NY: Readers Digest Association.

Greenberg, R. (1994, June/July). You can get insurance. *PWA Newsline, 5.*

Merson, M. H. (1994). *HIV/AIDS: The global epidemic and the global response.* Washington, DC: World Health Organization.

Pritchett, J. (Ed.). (1991). *The HIV/AIDS book: Information for workers* (4th ed.). Washington, DC: Occupational Health & Safety Department, Service Employees International Union.

South, K. (1993). AIDS and national health care reform. *New Conversations, 15,* 2.

Terl, A. (1992, February/March). Life insurance buyouts. *PWA Newsline,* 1–12.

Turnbull, L. (1992, October 21). AIDS patients' money worries eased. *The Beacon Journal,* pp. A1, A12.

U.S. Department of Health and Human Services. (1993). *A guide to Social Security and SSI Disability Benefits for people with HIV infection* (SSA Publication No. 05-10020). Washington, DC: U.S. Government Printing Office.

6

Living Together:
Challenges and Opportunities

Home, home, sweet, sweet home! There's no place like home! There's no place like home! —John Howard Payne (1791–1852)

This chapter addresses the need for and types of residential facilities, residents' expectations, staff training emphasizing cultural competency, tuberculosis and chemical dependency, volunteers, volunteer training, death, loss and grief issues, and memorialization. It will show how it is possible for health professionals from outside agencies to provide HIV/AIDS education and support to prison inmates. As HIV/AIDS has touched the lives of more and more individuals, so has the need for residential facilities grown.

Some infected people who desperately needed housing were already among the ranks of the homeless, but many more found themselves reduced to poverty through their inability to continue to work because of the progress of signs, symptoms, and opportunistic infections. Job loss frequently meant the loss of income, health insurance, and the ability to meet basic survival needs.

Poverty-stricken people come from all ethnic, educational, and age groups. Some had no family support systems. Others have families, but those families for a variety of reasons are unable or unwilling to provide the care that is needed. Other support systems may have come from friends who are now dead from the disease. Infected prison inmates often have nowhere to go when they are released. For years, nursing homes and adult congregate living facilities refused to admit people with AIDS. Through intensive staff education programs that picture has somewhat changed in some areas of the country, but there will always be those who will need a residential setting rather than the skilled and more confined services that are provided by nursing homes.

The number of infected women, children, and adolescents continues to climb, increasing the need for adequate, comprehensive, sensitive, and age-related facilities that cater to both sexes and include children under the age of 18.

RESIDENTIAL FACILITIES

In the early and mid-1980s, the need first arose for alternative housing for those who were unable to continue to support or care for themselves. Many grass-roots HIV/AIDS organizations and volunteers welcomed the sick and dying into their homes. Agencies rented houses in residential neighborhoods and provided care to several people under one roof. Neighborhoods did not always respond kindly to this arrangement, and the agencies were sometimes forced to close the houses and move the residents elsewhere. Since these early days, residential facilities have become more common, considerably less feared, and a lot more funded.

Residential facilities can range from foster homes; apartment complexes run by a trained, caring manager; adult congregate living facilities (ACLFs); small houses; and larger residences. They may provide subsidized rent and independent living in an apartment complex, assistance with daily living in an ACLF, or 24-hour-a-day child care in a foster home. Depending on their availability in the local area, they can be an enormous benefit, allowing families to stay together.

The Need

Deciding on what is needed means conducting a detailed survey of your community by contacting all of the AIDS service programs, the public health department, and local city and county authorities to find out what is currently being provided, where the gaps are, what is perceived to be needed now and in the future, and how to fill these gaps. Find out if there are any funding sources or available grants to assist a housing program. In South Florida, for example, funding for a variety of alternative housing programs has come from Ryan White monies, Community Foundation Grants, other local grants, and from the residents themselves when they are receiving Social Security benefits or other income that help to pay for their room and board.

State and Local Laws

Before starting this major commitment, find out what the pertinent legal issues are. For instance, how many beds are allowed without state licensure? Is an occupancy license required? What sort of zoning laws exist in the area that is being contemplated? Is there an existing available facility that already has the required license?

The Location

How will the neighborhood receive an HIV/AIDS facility in its midst? One of our larger residential facilities, before its inception, invited its proposed neighbors from a three-block radius to a community evening gathering. The group was told of the plans and invited to ask questions, make comments, and have their concerns addressed.

Much discussion occurred around the issue of HIV transmission, and many fears and myths were disclosed. Those fears and myths were apparently answered effectively, as there has never been a single problem; the neighborhood community is supportive and responsive to the program.

Transportation

There should be easy access to public transportation systems. Bus stops need to be nearby as long walks in bad weather can be exhausting. Link up with a community program that already provides transportation for persons with AIDS (PWAs). Encourage volunteers to assist with transportation needs.

THE RESIDENTS

Residents come from all walks of life. They come because they have no other means of support, do not want the support they do have, or are attempting to live on very slender means or no money at all. They may also be trying to get away from stigmatization, abusive relationships, and their own inability to continue to cope. They may recently have been released from prison and have nowhere else to turn. They may be young children who have lost both parents to AIDS and are now orphaned and alone.

Resident Expectations

Residents expect to receive protection, food, shelter, and companionship. They expect that someone will understand their needs and try to meet those needs whether they are emotional, spiritual, or physical.

Resident's Reality

Until one lives in a group setting, it is hard to understand that living together takes desire, commitment, and continuing effort. Residents give up freedom, privacy, and confidentiality. They may be required to sign away their financial resources and to receive in return a small weekly or monthly allowance. They are casting their lot among strangers from different social, cultural, ethnic, and behavioral backgrounds and at the same time are dealing with their own challenging issues. Sharing a room and a roof takes hard work and a forgiving spirit!

The Adjustment Process

The adjustment process is helped if the resident-to-be has a pretty good understanding of what to expect from the staff, physical amenities, payment requirements, and day-to-day rules and regulations before making the decision to move in.

When the individual does move in, his or her orientation should include an introduction to roommates and a daily schedule that assigns a time to meet as many of the staff as possible. Don't forget to introduce the housekeeping and kitchen employees. They often provide the homely link that the individual badly needs right now.

A written pamphlet is always useful. It can give the times that meals are served; the time of morning and night when the main doors are opened and closed; where there are soft drinks and snacks available; when the kitchen is closed; when residential council meetings are held; when other meetings are held; transportation schedules; the names, positions, and offices of the staff; important telephone numbers; and the location of HIV/AIDS medical clinics.

Resident's Council

Right from the inception of the program, make certain that the residents and the staff meet on a regular basis. A lot of unnecessary problems can be avoided, minimized, or resolved when residents and staff have an opportunity to discuss issues together. The residents perceive that they have influence, and the staff more readily understand the issues. It is a good idea to appoint a chairperson, take minutes, and keep the minutes in a looseleaf three-ring binder where they are easily available to the residents and staff.

STAFF EDUCATION AND TRAINING

This should be provided to all members of the staff by an educator who is knowledgeable in human behaviors and the current treatment and therapies for HIV/AIDS. Areas that should be covered include interpersonal communication and listening skills; cultural awareness; sexually transmitted diseases; signs, symptoms, prevention, and treatment for pulmonary tuberculosis; nutrition and nutritional supplements; chemical dependence; local resources; available support groups; medical advocacy; dying and death; grief and bereavement; developmental phases of childhood and adolescence; and pain and symptom management. Education needs to be a regular and ongoing part of the organizational structure.

Some of these topics are covered in other chapters, but it is appropriate to spend a little time discussing cultural competency, tuberculosis, and chemical dependence, as all of them affect residential facilities in the way that care is delivered.

Helping anyone means that there is a need to have some knowledge regarding cultural values and norms and an ability to be sensitive to other people's standards and belief systems. Ignorance of other people's belief systems and backgrounds frequently devalues the individual, prevents the development of trust, and negatively impacts the benefit and outcome of counseling.

CULTURAL AWARENESS

Everyone has some cultural differences from one another even when a common language is shared. We reflect the heritage of our birth country and family and interpret that heritage through education, religion, belief systems, values, taboos, skills, customs, institutions, ceremonies, national pastimes, and politics.

Sue and Sue's (1990) extremely informative book *Counseling the Culturally Different* quoted Pederson, who noted, "U.S. culture and society is based upon the concept of individualism and that competition between individuals for status, recognition, achievement, and so forth, forms the basis for Western tradition" (p. 35). Pederson also stated that

> *not all cultures view individualism as a positive orientation; rather, it may be perceived in some cultures as a handicap to attaining enlightenment, one that may divert us from important spiritual goals. In many non-western cultures identity is not seen apart from the group orientation. (p. 35)*

Westerners themselves come in wonderfully different shapes, sizes, and colors, and each one reflects his or her own unique history verbally, psychosocially, emotionally, and behaviorally. Discomfort is often felt when someone of a different race responds in a different way to our own self-imposed and expected stereotypes. So often this stereotype is the tragic seed that produces discrimination for no other reason than a difference in appearance, expression, or economic status.

To effectively counsel those from different backgrounds requires desire, openness, enlightenment, acceptance, and a broadening of skills that encourages the development of compatible goals appropriate to the client's needs.

Enlightenment comes through a genuine and ongoing wish to understand other people's values. As understanding and knowledge grow, so too will relevant and effective goals be attained. Cross-cultural understanding is an immeasurably powerful and beautiful experience from which everyone wins. Don't be afraid to venture into these uncharted waters because there are all sorts of extraordinary places to explore.

People communicate in several ways, some of which are explained here.

Nonverbal Communication

Nonverbal communication includes silence, distance, eye contact, body movements, and emotional expressiveness.

Silence. Silence in 20th-century America seems to have practically disappeared. Car radios rock other cars with their decibel levels, elevators fill our ears with canned music, computerized telephone services blast us with words and song, and conversation never seems to be allowed a pause for thought or reflection. Even places of worship are frequently full of chatter and noise. Other cultures may enjoy long periods of silence or, conversely, find it perfectly normal to speak before the other person has finished. Learn about the appropriate use of pauses and interruptions in other cultures and abide by them. Disrupting silence may cause the client to completely retreat and waste a precious opportunity for trust, understanding, and communication that may never reoccur.

Distance or proximity. There is not one of us who at some time has not felt discomfited when someone has thrust his or nose 2 inches from ours, "in our face," and spoken loudly at us and not to us. There is an instinctive move to step back or push them away. But cultures differ. Generally, and there are exceptions to all norms, Anglos tend to keep people at arms' length or shaking-hands distance, Asians prefer a greater distance, and Latin Americans, French, West Indians, Black Americans, South Americans, and Arabs usually prefer a closer distance. How close is comfortable may also be dictated by class, social stature, gender, wealth, and individual personality. The appropriate distance can be a veritable little minefield, so be cautious. Ask clients where they would like to sit. Some will prefer counselors to stay safely behind their desks so that there is visual separation, others will prefer to be within touching distance, yet others prefer to be side by side. Asking clients where they would like to sit and noting their subsequent choices will help to indicate their preference in matters of distance.

Eye contact. Most Anglos want others to look them squarely in the eye in the belief (often mistaken) that this portrays trustworthiness, honesty, and a look into the soul of the individual. If people don't do this, they are frequently regarded as shifty, dishonest, sullen, uncooperative, and rude. Black Americans may regard eye contact as disrespectful when listening but when speaking often make greater eye contact than Anglos. Asians and Native Americans may see eye contact as hostile and impolite. Watch your client for clues as to what, if any, eye contact is acceptable.

Body movements or kinesics. Body movements include laughter and smiling, head shaking, posture, gestures, and facial expressions. Body movements are strongly linked to cultural background, and misinterpretation of these movements can alter the assessment and cause unintentional misunderstandings. Britons are brought up as pragmatists with a stiff upper lip; Asians are taught to restrain strong feelings such as anger, sadness, and happiness as this restraint reflects maturity; Native Americans find vigorous hand shaking aggressive, whereas Latin Americans shake hands energetically and Anglos use hand shaking as a method of introduction, good will, and pleasure at seeing another. Some are "must" huggers. Strangers or friends will be indiscriminately clutched to the bosom. This is just not OK for everyone. Be observant of body movements, and when you are uncertain ask your client. Clients much prefer honesty and are usually only too willing to fill in the cultural gaps.

Emotional expressiveness. Not everyone will express themselves emotionally. They may display no tears, sorrow, laughter, pain, or joy. They may become labeled as less intelligent, inarticulate, unrealistic, passive, and antagonistic. What a disservice is done to them! Intimate problems may not be discussed because they reflect not only on the individual but on the family. This is particularly so in Asian societies. Hispanics and American Indians may reflect similar values.

Black Americans may not see a White counselor as one who understands their issues, but rather as a busybody who may not keep their affairs confidential. The counselor may be seen as a parent figure, which leaves the client in a subordinate role even though this is not the intention. Understanding that emotional expressiveness is different within cultures and personalities and discussing this with clients will help to promote ease and comprehension for both client and counselor.

Verbal Communication

Counseling is very much a process of accurately interpreting the words, thoughts, needs, and goals of the client. Many of us in the West speak only standard

English, which places those who speak either nonstandard English or a different primary language at a definite disadvantage.

Counselors need to remember that volume of voice, soft or loud, is more indicative of one's cultural background than of anger, hostility, weakness, shyness, or depression. For instance, loud voices are normal for some cultures such as Arabs and North Americans, but Asians tend to use softer voices. Tune into the individual's speech volume and pattern and speak using similar tones.

Euphemisms and ambiguity may be normal, and "opening up," on which we Westerners place such enormous value, may be embarrassing and societally unacceptable. Practical advice may be far more important to the client than an explanation of deeper feelings, which may be seen as interfering and inappropriate.

Expressing one's own thoughts, feelings, hopes, and challenges can develop a level of trust that may not have occurred without some thoughtful self-disclosures from the counselor. This may include identifying and discussing the differences that appear to exist between the client and the counselor and a mutual agreement that it is worth trying to understand these differences.

Counselors will often succeed when they are willing to be flexible, open, honest, and educated. Failure occurs when they refuse to address their own racial and cultural beliefs, which may be absolutely contrary to the client's beliefs and value systems.

What a dull, colorless world it would be if we looked, talked, cried, ate, drank, and communicated in the same way! Diversity should not be scary but a wonderful opportunity to add education, wisdom, and harmony to the very fabric of our own lives.

Counselors who find themselves counseling different cultures should explore those cultures in any way possible through language classes, libraries, documentaries regarding the client's country of birth, and culturally aware travel books such as the *Lonely Planet* and *Travelers World* guidebooks. Clients are usually thrilled when they find that their counselor has taken the time to find out something about their historical background and to offer a few phrases, however unusually pronounced, in their birth language. Sharing recipes and food opens up doors of communication and understanding that are impossible to overstate.

Effective communication is the key to preventing transmission, accessing information, increasing support, encouraging enrollment in research programs, maintaining medication regimens, allowing feedback, developing support systems, validating needs, exploring feelings, and providing a continuum of efficient and compassionate care.

Cultural communication may be hazardous and misunderstood, but perseverance and a genuine desire to be nonjudgmental will frequently reap a beautiful and productive harvest.

TUBERCULOSIS

There has been a resurgence of tuberculosis (TB) throughout the United States. "When people with HIV or AIDS are exposed to TB they have the same risk of becoming infected as individuals not exposed to HIV" (Jones & Tynan, 1994, p. 1).

Individuals who have carried a harmless TB infection around for years very often develop active TB not long after becoming HIV+ (Stead, 1992). The crowded conditions typically seen in residential facilities such as jails, congregate living facilities, and shelters for the homeless increase the risk of exposure to TB. Individuals who are HIV+ have an immune system that is now more vulnerable to TB.

The staffs of residential facilities need to determinedly attempt to reduce the risk of TB transmission to other residents and to themselves. TB is an airborne disease but will not usually be transmitted to another person unless there is prolonged exposure. One of the requirements to consider for a residential facility is whether to screen all applicants for TB before admission. If they test positive for TB, a decision should then be made as to where they will receive their initial treatment and whether they must wait to be admitted to the facility until they are no longer infectious.

Whatever decisions are made, certain things still need to occur. All residents should be screened once a year; staff should be screened at least once a year; rooms should be well ventilated by using ceiling fans, opening windows, and installing individual air conditioning units in each bedroom; residents must take their medications as and when they are prescribed, and the staff should provide supervision and support; counseling should be ongoing for the infected residents and for their family members; other residents should receive TB prevention education; and staff and volunteers should receive ongoing TB training.

CHEMICAL DEPENDENCE

Residential facilities have found real challenges in the number of clients who use illicit drugs. For years, a number of facilities either refused to take in those who were actively using drugs, or threw the clients out when they were caught. Neither way was a very positive solution. Now many facilities have an on-site chemical dependency group that meets 5 days a week and is run by a certified addictions professional. The meetings help to stabilize this sometimes volatile population and reduce the incidents of relapse. Individual counseling is there if it is needed.

OCCUPATIONAL THERAPY

An occupational or recreational therapist can be a paid professional, a volunteer, or someone with the ability to encourage individuals into more creatively using their lives. It doesn't matter what title these individuals have, they are an essential part of this kind of program.

Residents should be encouraged to either use talents that they already have or find ones that they did not even know were there. We all have hidden gifts, and a sensitive, skilled therapist can find them. It could be learning to play cards, draw, paint, or create sand drawings or pottery, weave, do macrame, make a photographic memory book, write one's life story, create a poem, play a musical instrument, learn line dancing, develop a choir, keep a diary, read or listen to a book, get one's spiritual life in order, volunteer in programs outside the facility, and so on. The list is endless and the horizons limitless, but it does take an energetic, dedicated person to implement and maintain the program. A volunteer, or group of volunteers, may be delighted to offer their own talents to initiate the program.

VOLUNTEERS

Volunteers are a wonderful and caring resource who bring the element of home to the facility. Volunteers join for all sorts of reasons, often because they have lost someone that they loved to an opportunistic infection of AIDS or because they feel a real desire to give something back for all the blessings that they have in their own lives. All volunteers should be prescreened with a written questionnaire and a face-to-face interview. The questionnaire should identify who they are, why they want to volunteer, if they have had any recent major losses, what special talents or language skills they may have, if they have transportation, and when they are available. The face-to-face interview goes through the questionnaire in more depth. If a volunteer sees themselves as only giving and not receiving, be a little wary. These may be the ones who are burning with desire to save humanity and very often are those who fall by the wayside sooner rather than later. Others may be voyeuristic—they may want to see "what these people are really like"— and others, the huge majority who volunteer out of nonjudgmental love and compassion, are there because they want to be there and become an extraordinary and beautiful support to the entire program.

The reason for taking the loss history of the prospective volunteer is because if the volunteer has suffered a major loss during the previous year to 18 months, it may be best to wait before putting the volunteers with clients on a one-to-one basis. Some people genuinely believe that they will surmount their own grief by becoming involved and helping someone else. Grief is a process that takes time. Developing a relationship with other people who become more ill and die may powerfully confront them with the grief that they thought they were over. Taking the time to heal after a major loss is good for everyone's emotional health. These volunteers should be warmly welcomed to help with administrative tasks, serve meals, provide transportation, develop a speakers bureau, plan some special events, and organize fund-raisers.

Volunteer Training

A volunteer already brings energy, enthusiasm, and a generous heart. A good, basic orientation training program will provide them with some useful knowledge and skills, an understanding of the program, guidance, and direction.

Orientation and training should not be rushed. They should cover specific topics, taught by the best available educator, and be held either on weekends or in the evenings, particularly if the majority of those volunteering are working people.

Topics to Cover

Topics should include the philosophy, mission, and goals of the program; basic HIV/AIDS education; sensitivity training regarding HIV/AIDS; the role of the volunteer; cultural sensitivity; confidentiality; body mechanics; listening and communications skills; pastoral care; the role of the case manager; developmental stages of children; emotional aspects of adolescence dealing with a chronic illness; documentation; community resources; personal attitudes toward dying and death; women's issues; bereavement and grief; legal issues; advance directives; living wills; the role of Social Security in HIV/AIDS; stress management; and reminiscence and relaxation therapies. This list can be broadened or narrowed to become pertinent to the community that you serve, but it does provide some ideas.

Ongoing education, support, and recognition are the keys to retaining volunteers. Do remember that volunteers are truly priceless and should be treasured. They should be affirmed, thanked, and never overwhelmed, or one day they will no longer be there.

Use of Volunteers

Volunteers may bring professional skills that are invaluable. They may be nurses, lawyers, linguists, doctors, accountants, massage therapists, music therapists, contractors, seamstresses, electricians, plumbers, fund-raisers, journalists, or commercial vehicle drivers. Some may want to use their professional talents; others may prefer a complete change. Volunteers can listen; read; write letters for those who are no longer able to write; accompany clients to medical appointments; take them for a walk on the beach, an outing to a football or baseball game, an afternoon at the races, or a religious service; pick up medications; and provide transportation for other family members so that they can visit the client. The list is endless. Do remember that volunteers need some boundaries. The client may ask them to do things for which they feel either untrained or uncomfortable. Make sure that they know their limits and are OK about saying "Sorry, I'm not allowed to do that."

Volunteers can be used for fund-raising, a speakers bureau, and special events. They may type, file, answer telephones, photocopy, write thank-you letters for donations, keep volunteer time records, address and stuff envelopes, and attend to the many small details that help the administrative department to run more smoothly.

Volunteers should be seen by the paid staff as an integral part of the entire organization. They are special people who bring special talents quietly and unselfishly. Look after them!

Residential facilities for PWAs are there to meet identified needs. The staff who run them are usually made up of highly skilled, extraordinarily dedicated, motivated, and creative individuals. They give their very best 24 hours a day, 7 days a week.

Intellectually, the staff recognize that the majority of their clients will die sooner or later. The reality of this inevitable separation is usually not felt until death is either imminent or has occurred, at which time the staff's own grief becomes apparent.

LOSS AND GRIEF

The depth of the staff's grief for each individual will depend on the events surrounding the death, whether there was an opportunity to say goodbye, the relationship between the deceased and each individual, other concurrent events, and an employee's personal history of losses.

Events Surrounding the Death

When a person dies in pain, alone, in the middle of the night, either in the residential facility or in a hospital and possibly while still receiving intensive rehabilitative care, those of us who remain frequently ask ourselves if this was a death that could have been managed more humanely.

Relatives and friends may have wished to be at the bedside and were not called in time because that request was not known by the staff on duty. Someone may have dialed 911 and resuscitation procedures that the client may have specifically said, but not written, that they did not want may have been started. These events need not happen if a few simple steps are taken. Speaking with residents about their wishes surrounding dying and death when they are in a reasonably good state of health will clarify their desires. This ensures that everyone is prepared to institute the appropriate care that most accurately reflects clients' expressed wishes when they are no longer able to speak for themselves.

Advance directives documentation will give guidance to staff members, and each person who provides direct care should be aware of them. Relatives and friends should have their names and telephone numbers on the front of the client's chart. A note should be made against each name as to whether they wish to be present before and during the death process. If a person does not have a telephone, make certain to ask for a neighbor's number and record it. When anyone is called to come to the bedside of a dying patient, do remember to suggest that they ask someone else to drive them and to wait with them. However much they may be expecting the call, it will still be a painful and sad shock, and they should neither drive alone nor be left on their own. Don't call 911 unless there are no written orders regarding resuscitation. When someone is dying and then resuscitated, rushed to a hospital emergency department and then to an intensive care unit and invaded by high-tech equipment, it becomes an assault on their dignity and their ability to die comfortably surrounded by those who matter to them. It is unbelievably costly to their physical, emotional, spiritual, and financial well-being, and their relatives and friends suffer similarly. If only we could change our view that death is a failure and allow it to be a time of peaceful transition, how much better off the patient and his or her family and loved ones would be.

Saying Goodbye

When someone dies and we were separated by any kind of distance, how much we wish that we had shared a last thought, a smile, a prayer, or a silence together. A residential facility provides a wonderful opportunity to say goodbye because it is easy to stop in the room for a brief, shared moment of caring. People who are dying do need to be quiet and pain free, but they do not need to be isolated. We, because we are sometimes afraid of dying and death, frequently leave them alone. Impending death is truly not scary. If we allow ourselves time to sit beside them, touch their hands, and share our thoughts, it can be an experience of overwhelming growth and love. In talking with them, tell them who is present and let them know that everything is OK, that it is all right for them to move on. It is believed that hearing and touch are with us until the moment of death, so even if they appear to be unconscious, continue to talk to and hold them.

Goodbye Rituals

Not everyone will have had the occasion to see the person before death. There are several things that can still be done; these include, but are not limited to, the following.

Funeral and memorial service. Encourage staff and residents who were close to the deceased to attend the funeral or memorial service. Services validate the person's life, support family and friends, and allow grief to be shared in a safe environment.

Memorial books. Keep a large, parchment-leafed album, inscribed with the person's name, birth date, and death date. It can be arranged by month and year. A talented volunteer may be willing to start it and maintain it. It is very beautiful if it is inscribed in hand-lettered calligraphy, but if that is not possible there are some marvelous fonts available for computers that can produce many forms of lettering that look almost like the real thing.

Memorial books have a lot of meaning to friends and relatives, and remind us all of people who have made an impression on our lives. They can be displayed formally at appropriate events during the year and made available at any time. When they are displayed, be sure to have plenty of facial tissues nearby as tears often accompany the turning of the pages.

Memorial tree. A memorial tree can be created in any way that you like. It could be made from either plywood or construction paper and painted. It can be attached to the wall of a quiet room, a chapel, or wherever it feels right. Large, separate cut-out leaves can be attached with velcro, stuck, pinned, or hung onto it with the name of the person who died. Trees and leaves are wonderful symbols of the everlasting circle of life and symbolically witness the presence of those who are no longer physically with us.

Informal remembrance services. These can be held in a designated area indoors or outdoors and can be either at a regular time during the year or as frequently as is felt necessary. It is a good idea to appoint a pastoral care counselor to facilitate the service, and it should be appropriate to the person or persons being remembered. Photographs, favorite flowers, poems, readings from books, or a favorite piece of clothing are specific personal reminders. For example, a dear friend died earlier this year; he was never without his beat-up, much worn, dark brown, broad-brimmed Australian hat. It was an integral part of his character. At his memorial service, it rested on top of the piano, reminding each one of us of the precious and often funny memories that were part of his bequest to us. Services do not have to be long; everyone should have the opportunity to speak, sing, dance, or play a tribute if they want to. Grieving together is supportive and healthy.

Grief support meeting. Many grief counselors would be more than willing to facilitate a support meeting. Sometimes staff, particularly health professionals, need to be reminded that it is OK to grieve. We don't always have to be, nor should we be, competent and strong. Sometimes we must acknowledge and feel our loss. Continuing unexpressed losses will eventually become overwhelming and can lead to the dreaded burn-out.

Groups can be held regularly once a month or meet whenever there seems to be the need. The facilitator can distribute handouts that describe the feelings and phases of grief and bereavement and offer some ideas for intervention that revolve around the need to be gentle to oneself and to recognize that all of us will grieve at one time or another.

Last, it is important that people play, particularly when their job, enjoyable as it may be, has built-in stressors. Sometimes just leaving the facility and strolling round the block will relieve tension, but other times more formal excursions such as a picnic on the beach or a visit to Disneyland provide the opportunity to have fun and learn a lot more about one's coworkers.

Working and living in a residential facility is a challenging experience. Known lifestyle, behaviors, and family systems may have completely changed. The quality of such a facility relies on the training, skills, empathy, and attentiveness brought to it by its staff and the willingness of the individual resident to cooperate, negotiate, and nonjudgmentally support the others. The following is a discussion of less obvious and talked-about residential facilities: federal, state, and county prisons.

EDUCATION AND SUPPORT FOR PRISON INMATES

Six years ago, the superintendent of one of Florida's state maximum security women's prisons asked me if I would consider organizing some HIV/AIDS sensitivity training programs for inmates, prison officers, and the health staff. She told me that she had come to me because prisoners who were either believed to be or known to be HIV+ or in full-blown AIDS were being subjected to all sorts of harassment. They were frequently verbally and sometimes physically abused by their fellow prisoners. Their lockers were ripped open and their personal belongings either stolen or destroyed. They were undesirable as "bunkies" (sharing the same dormitory space) as there was real fear that they would and could pass the dreaded virus along. Basic HIV/AIDS education was a mandatory part of every inmate's life, but the emotional, psychological, and spiritual issues associated with the retrovirus were given little or no attention.

It was remarkable and exciting to me to find that the chief advocate for HIV-infected inmates was the head of that particular institution. It was her sensitivity, enthusiasm, and commitment that started a program that is now one of three models being used by the State of Florida to establish similar projects statewide.

Although I thought that the sensitivity training program was a great idea, I still approached it with a sense of trepidation. The penal system was virtually unknown to me. I felt that punishment rather than rehabilitation was the system's prime focus and that inmates themselves could be very intimidating. However, the challenge beckoned.

THE BEGINNING

It was agreed that each of the seven dormitories would receive a mandatory sensitivity training program of 2–3 hours duration delivered over the course of 7 consecutive weeks. Each dormitory houses 100 inmates of varying ages and ethnic and cultural backgrounds.

The Program

Sessions were held in the facility's very large gym. Seats were arranged in orderly rows, and prison officers stood behind and at the sides of the rows. This, as can be imagined, was not exactly conducive to the sharing of thoughts and feelings! The superintendent started off each meeting by explaining why the participants were there, some of the negative events that had occurred on the compound, that HIV/AIDS was not going to go away, and that the number of infected prisoners was increasing. She told the audience who I was and that she hoped that the program would help to change some of their attitudes regarding the virus and their neighbors. She encouraged everyone to ask questions and to address their fears, beliefs, and thoughts.

At each session, a video entitled *Mother, Mother* (Dickoff & Praiser, 1989), which told the story of an HIV-infected young man and his relationship with his mother, was shown. It is very moving and tapped into a lot of emotions. Handkerchiefs, facial tissues, and paper towels were much in evidence as it was shown. Afterwards, the comments and questions came fast and furiously. Somehow we quickly established a rapport and the beginnings of a mutual trust that is evident to this day.

I answered questions as honestly as possible. The superintendent had already suggested and authorized an HIV/AIDS support group. This was an excellent opportunity to tell this to the inmates, who were advised to start sharing information and receiving support when the sensitivity training sessions were completed.

The following week, a gorgeous, outspoken, and humorous HIV-infected man— Roger, to whom this book is dedicated—came along. The inmates loved him. They were as frank with him as he was with them, and it was possible to literally see negative attitudes changing.

During the 7 weeks of the program, we were often blessed by Roger's cheerful and articulate presence, and as the inmates opened up more and more my own commitment to developing an ongoing HIV/AIDS support group grew.

Results of Sensitivity Training

Those who were infected reported that no more nasty incidents had occurred since the sessions had started, and although some people would still not have very much to do with them, the verbal abuse had almost stopped. There was still a long way to go, but the prognosis seemed a lot more hopeful than it had been 2 months earlier and the time appeared to be right to start the HIV/AIDS support group.

THE HIV/AIDS SUPPORT GROUP

Personnel

The superintendent assigned a member of the psychosocial department to be the designated prison official at each meeting. That individual was responsible for seeing that the inmates knew where and when the group met, meeting and escorting me to the room, attending every session, keeping informal notes as to subject matter, providing accurate interpretation of prison rules, identifying health delivery changes as they occurred, and encouraging infected or affected inmates to attend. This individual needed to be realistic, compassionate, trusted, and informed. Our group is extraordinarily blessed by having a young woman who is all of the above, as well as steadfast, gentle, and dedicated. She has played a crucial role in the program's success.

The Group

The group meets every other Friday afternoon from 2:00 to 3:30 P.M. in a room in the Educational Building. Attendance is voluntary, participation is voluntary, and it is an open group. Some of the original members still attend today, others have left, and others come once every 2, 3, or 6 months.

In the beginning, the group was very small, with no more than 5 or 6 attendees. The low attendance apparently was because people were terrified to be seen coming to an HIV support group and were afraid of renewed stigmatization. By the end of the first year, it had grown to about 12 members and now numbers 15–20 members.

The first months were ones of developing trust, seeing who was going to take control (the group or me!), and storms of griping, particularly at conditions in the infirmary over which I neither had nor intended to have any kind of power to intervene.

At this time in the group's evolution, we reached consensus on a short list of group rules that are as follows.

Group Rules

Confidentiality. This rule addressed confidentiality between inmate and inmate, inmate and staff, staff and inmate, inmate and me, and me and inmate. This is emphasized at every session. It is explained that sharing someone else's story outside of the group may cause needless harmful gossip, leading to the destruction of trust within the group.

If something is said that suggests one of the participants is thinking seriously about committing suicide, she is reminded that the psychosocial worker cannot keep this confidential and must tell the medical staff, which will result in the individual being removed from her dormitory and being placed under a suicide watch.

If a particular issue is to be presented to the superintendent, consensus is reached by the entire group and then presented from the group without mentioning individual names.

Timeliness. People are asked to start and leave on time as a courtesy to each other.

Permission. A written pass is needed to attend the group.

Speaking. One person speaks at a time, and people are discouraged from speaking for the entire session. There is a "no-more-than-3-minutes" rule; however, adherence is rare.

Intent. The group is intended to be supportive, empathetic, and educational, not to be a prolonged listing of woes. Occasionally every misery, perceived or real, is ventilated, but these sessions are now rare.

Supporting each other. One of the reasons why people attend is to receive support from the facilitator and from each other. Support is truly given and received when it is offered nonjudgmentally, regardless of the quantity or quality of the need or the personality and values of the recipient.

Touching. Touching within the prison is forbidden. I do give hugs within the privacy of the room when they seem appropriate. Ignoring the prison rules and causing contretemps could cause the cessation of the group.

If you are considering working within the correctional system and are new to the system, make certain that you obtain and read the rules before commencing. Study them carefully, and if you have any questions ask for answers beforehand.

Facilitator's Rules

I have very few facilitator's rules; they are self-imposed and work for me. You will establish ones that work for you. I never, ever ask why an individual is incarcerated. Originally this occurred because I was aware that many of the inmates' crimes were related to first- and second-degree murder, and I was not sure how I would mentally handle this. Would I become judgmental, afraid, or discriminatory? Later, it seemed an intrusion to ask. Sometimes it is volunteered. One of the surprises was that very few people protest their innocence.

Dress to the teeth! At the inception of the program, the administrator of a community-based HIV organization told me I'd "better dress down and dirty." I looked puzzled, and she elaborated by saying that I needed to be just like the inmates to develop trust. I believed that this attitude devalued the inmates and made me a poor role model. Feedback from the inmates is that I bring class, style, and a sense of the outside world.

Self-disclose when it seems appropriate. For instance, I spent some of my teenage years attending boarding school and then lived for 5 years under the stringent rule of a British nursing school. Twelve-hour shifts were the order of the day and night, we were allowed late-night passes (allowed out until 11:00 p.m.) twice a month in our second year, the food was canteen-style, and nearly every move we made was critically watched. Just so that we did not become attached to our bedroom, we were arbitrarily moved every 3 months. None of this is meant to be compared with a life of incarceration, but it did teach me a great deal about learning to live with strangers, all of whom were women.

Share photos. Many of the inmates have children, and we are able to share some of our experiences and outcomes. Bringing in photographs of vacations is always welcomed, but screen family snapshots taken at home for identifiers. One inmate recognized my condominium building, and retrospectively it seems a good idea not to show personal locales that could be recognized.

Follow prison rules. Don't promise anything you cannot deliver, and don't get into a confrontational situation with the system. Recognize special holidays by giving cards, but find out the rules. At our prison, cards can be brought in, but the envelopes must be left unsealed.

Establishing some simple rules for the group and for yourself helps to develop guidelines, establish boundaries, and promote cohesion.

The curricula for the program originally focused on the psychosocial issues surrounding HIV/AIDS, and these issues remain the underlying theme. However, as we have become more familiar with each other, the contents of the program have broadened.

Group Content

At the beginning of each calendar year, the group is invited to suggest the programs it would like to have. They include the opportunistic infections of AIDS; signs, symptoms, and treatment; losses attached to HIV; AIDS dementia; nursing care of terminally ill persons; stress management; expressing anger without ending up in "lock-up"; current affairs; legal issues of advance directives, living wills, and wills; Social Security, Medicare, and Medicaid; listening skills; the how-tos of effective communication; acute and chronic pain management; tuberculosis; diabetes; reminiscence therapy; grief and bereavement; coping with holidays; relaxation therapy; guided imagery; self-massage; external resources; reconciliation and forgiveness; and the 3-minute stress manager.

Some expected and unexpected outcomes have occurred during the past 6 years.

EXPECTED OUTCOMES

One of the original objectives was to change the negative attitudes and behaviors of the inmates toward those who were infected with HIV. There has been a marked change, and no longer are there occurrences of the nasty events of the late 1980s. Furthermore, many of the uninfected inmates have become knowledgeable, supportive, and actively helpful to the infected inmates.

Inservices were given to the medical staff on HIV/AIDS treatment, emphasizing the emotional issues in particular. This, combined with a much more aggressive policy toward prophylactic intervention and better use of medications for opportunistic infections, has raised the standard of care.

Within the group, behaviors generally improved. Aggression and overt hostility lessened, and stressors are managed more appropriately, resulting in less time being confined to solitary in lock-up (which is jocularly referred to as the Hotel Hilton).

UNEXPECTED OUTCOMES

Two of the unexpected outcomes at this particular prison were the development
of a nursing assistance program to help those hospitalized in the infirmary and
around-the-clock visitation of patients designated as terminally ill. The visitation
program started when one of the group became extremely ill with a brain tumor,
was barely able to move, and complained of soul-destroying loneliness. The superintendent was asked if people could be permitted to visit. She said yes, under
the proviso that they were regular group members, that they had an understanding
of the dying process, and that the patient had identified whom she would like to
visit her. As everyone wanted to be part of the roster, there were some feelings of
rejection when she named whom she wanted to see. These feelings were worked
through during the group sessions.

The visitation program continued successfully for several years. Then people
expressed a desire to have some basic nursing skills such as making beds; giving a
bed bath; helping with a bed pan; transferring a person from bed to a commode,
wheelchair, or bathroom; assisting with showers; and feeding someone who could
no longer feed herself.

By this time, another nurse had volunteered her time to work with the group so
vacations could be taken without stopping the meetings. She has proven to be
marvelous. We have very different personalities and so bring to the group our
own unique qualities. She developed and implemented the nursing assistance program, wrote a training manual, and holds regular training sessions, as well as
running the regular sessions with particular emphasis on diseases, disease process,
treatment, and care.

Another unexpected outcome is the provision of interdisciplinary hospice services to those inmates who meet the hospice criteria and request the program.
This has improved pain and symptom management and the delivery of care to the
dying.

Individual counseling is given to those who request it. They may be in the
infirmary and want to talk about their lives, their hopes, their needs, and their
fears, or they may want to discuss issues that they do not wish to address during
the group meeting. Recently, a young woman whose mother was dying from cancer asked for individual counseling. The inmate received permission to go and see
her for 2 weeks in the custody of the sheriff from her small rural hometown.
Although she desperately wanted to go, she was extremely afraid of how other
members of her family, the sheriff, and townspeople would treat her. We role-
played a worst-case scenario of rejection by her family, friends, and townspeople.
When she felt fairly comfortable with the possibility of rejection, she was able to
leave feeling nervous but not terrified. The visit was sad because of her mother's
deterioration but wonderful because she was, without exception, treated with kind-
ness and understanding.

It became possible not only to provide outside HIV/AIDS resources for the
time when people have completed their sentences but also to place them in residential facilities when there were no other support systems. One young woman
became a resident and not too long afterwards complained of seeing brightly colored flashing lights. As soon as it could be arranged, she was examined by an

ophthalmologist who diagnosed cytomegalovirus (CMV) in both eyes. From my point of view, it was imperative that she begin treatment with gangcyclovir as soon as possible to try to prevent further deterioration. The protocol was explained to her, and she adamantly refused. Her explanation was that she had spent the past 10 years in prison and she was not going to be imprisoned again by intravenous therapy. Her reasoning was very understandable, but it was very hard to see her sight slowly disappear until she decided that she would commence the regimen, which came far too late. She loved to paint and at the last she was quite blind, unable to see paint, brush, or paper. Honoring someone's desires is not always easy.

After a couple of years, the state said that it was discriminatory to call the support group an HIV/AIDS support group, and it became a support group for those affected by a chronic illness. In 1995, the state mandated that all prisons have an HIV/AIDS support group, and ours will be used as one of the role models. However, a number of those infected have said that they want to stay with this group—we continue our process of evolution!

EVOLUTION

Recent comments by the group participants regarding the benefits that they have derived from attending included the following: "The group provides normality; I can be myself and no one tells me that I have to be otherwise. In the prison we are castrated from normal life." "I really love it when your Mom visits." "I've learned to accept that some things cannot be changed." "Supporting someone else is nurturing to me." "Comforting." "Sharing. In the group, for a short while I'm not in a fish bowl." "Encouragement." "Developing friends who support me." "Humanizing." "Accepting others and putting self aside."

My mother is 89, lives in England, and comes to Ft. Lauderdale for Christmas every year. She visits the group at least once each time and is truly loved. She is mother, grandmother, and great-grandmother to them. She is not a "touchy-feely" person, but she visibly values them and they value her. She brings news of the British royal family, British history, winter storms, her garden, and her volunteer work. She refers to the group when she is back home as "my dear friends" and regularly corresponds with them, sending newspaper clippings and booklets about historical landmarks and things of interest. She too brings normality and is a powerful role model of gentleness, caring, and sharing.

THE FACILITATOR

To make an HIV/AIDS support group work, it is essential to have the support of the superintendent and, if possible, that of the medical director. The internal person who is assigned to the group needs to welcome the project and be willing to act as the conduit between the group and the administrative staff.

An effective facilitator should have a sense of humor, be nonjudgmental and almost shock-proof, have a sound knowledge of HIV/AIDS issues, be aware of the penal code and rules, act as a role model, have the ability to self-disclose appropriately, interact comfortably with the prison staff, and understand and value cultural and socioeconomic differences.

Find out if you can take in candy and cookies. This not only gives everyone an afternoon glucose high but provides a moment of sharing food that invariably results in feeling good.

The group has become a cohesive unit of individuals who look out for each other and bring something unique to every one of us. Running a prison group is challenging but has far-reaching rewards.

CONCLUSION

The need for a variety of residential facilities for the housing of people infected with HIV/AIDS will continue to grow in the foreseeable future. The staff of these facilities will need to be experienced in both clinical knowledge and their ability to create a pleasant homelike setting and atmosphere. They will frequently serve people whose lifestyles have placed them at risk, and they will need to be nonjudgmental but have the ability to establish comprehensive boundaries. Residential facilities provide a wonderful opportunity to give care and support to those who no longer are able to do that for themselves.

If it is possible, clients should be allowed to complete their lives in the facility, surrounded by the people and things that are known to them. Staff will need to grieve, whatever position they hold. The signs and symptoms of burnout should be recognized, and intervention should occur sooner rather than later.

Prison systems show an increasing number of infected inmates. The well-being of those who are infected and affected can be enhanced by the development of educational and emotional support groups that may also lead to the development of other programs.

REFERENCES

Dickoff, M., & Praiser, I. (Producers). (1989). *Mother, Mother* [Videotape]. Los Angeles: AIDS Hospice Foundation.

Jones, M. J., & Tynan, E. J. (Eds). (1994). TB and HIV. Tuberculosis adds to the challenge of the epidemic. *AIDS Information Exchange, 11*(2).

Stead, W. W. (1992). *Understanding tuberculosis today.* (8th ed.). Milwaukee, WI: Central Press.

Sue, W. S., & Sue, D. (1990). *Counseling the culturally different.* New York: John Wiley & Sons.

7

The Spiritual Dimension

Spirituality is a process we must each define for ourselves. It involves learning to live in the moment, valuing being over accomplishment, finding connection with something greater than ourselves, and accepting all of ourselves—both good and bad.
—Regina Renteria (1995)

This chapter is not about individual religions or morality. It is more of an attempt to look at the things that deter us from becoming whole, spontaneous, joyful, and integrated beings and suggests ways that may assist with that integration or reintegration.

THE RELIGIOUS COMMUNITY

The formal religious bodies have taken an enormous length of time in addressing HIV/AIDS within their communities. Those institutions lost many opportunities in the 1980s to preach and practice nonjudgmental love, HIV prevention, and support to affected and infected individuals. Instead, the majority of religious leaders either turned their backs on the virus and hoped that it would go away or wallowed in apathy and did nothing. A few preached hellfire and damnation from the pulpit and the airwaves, assuring those who were infected that this disease was God's will and they deserved what they got. Priest, pastors, rabbis, ministers, and congregations were often uncomfortable when AIDS came to them.

A Reform Jewish woman's husband died from the opportunistic infections of AIDS several years ago. She kept this a secret from her temple but desperately wanted to tell the congregation the truth. She went to her rabbi and said that she wished to share her story. The rabbi was stunned by her news and eventually said to her "I'm OK with the truth but I know that the congregation is not yet ready." She left him feeling that he was the one who was not ready. Neither of them have ever addressed the issue again, and HIV/AIDS remains a buried secret between them. This has caused her to question her religious values and beliefs and to seek spiritual support elsewhere.

On another occasion, a young man who had just been released from a hospital after attempting suicide on a local beach came for counseling. He said that his father had thrown him out of the house when he learned of his son's homosexuality and HIV status. His mother was forbidden to write or speak to him. His father was a minister, as was his sister's husband. They all lived in another state. He and his counselor agreed that his family situation couldn't get much worse if they were contacted once again, and that there was everything to gain and not a lot to lose. He hoped there would be a change of heart and an invitation to return home, which is what he most wanted. The counselor placed the phone call and received a torrent of abuse from his father and brother-in-law about his lifestyle, behaviors, and unworthiness. She was told in no uncertain terms by his father that he had disowned his son who must never darken his doorstep again.

So many people shared similar experiences that it was truly heartening to find that in our midst there were three wonderful examples of religious leadership: a Baptist minister who started an HIV/AIDS ecumenical support group in a young, upwardly mobile parish and wrote one of the first church-inspired books on HIV/AIDS (Amos, 1988); the Metropolitan Community Church whose congregation provided and continues to provide a positive cornucopia of services to the HIV-affected and -infected; and a Roman Catholic priest who has devoted many years to developing a thrift shop, food bank, and support systems for anyone who needs assistance regardless of their need, sex, age, religious, or cultural background.

At long last, there is a caring, religiously based nationwide network called the AIDS National Interfaith Network (ANIN) whose mission is to "link people of faith, mobilize religious leadership, promote quality pastoral care, encourage culturally appropriate prevention education, and foster provision of compassionate, non-judgmental services to and advocacy on behalf of those infected and affected by HIV/AIDS" (South, 1994, p. 1).

The network is rapidly expanding its membership, and many faiths are represented. At a local level, there are a growing number of HIV pastoral care networks that interface with HIV community-based programs, educate religious leaders, advocate for religious and spiritual care, visit infected and affected persons, build friendships and coalitions, seek funding, and discourage intolerance and bigotry. The national office of ANIN can tell you if there is a local program near you.

When Cicely Saunders started the modern-day hospice movement in the 1960s, she believed that the individual and his or her attendant family suffered from a variety of pains, including spiritual pain. Spiritual pain is unique to each of us. Many of us have had, have, or will have spiritual pain in our lives regardless of whether we are physically healthy or sick.

SPIRITUAL PAIN

Many health professionals tend to disregard the spiritual and religious dimensions of their patients and clients. Denying or ignoring the complex and multifaceted issues that face those infected and affected by HIV may be refusing them the opportunity to legitimize their pain and to work through their fears, anxieties, values, and beliefs, which could lead to forgiveness, personal growth, reconciliation, and resolution.

There are those clients who may have no religious affiliation but who still search for meaning and understanding. Our task is to recognize their pain, to provide avenues that lead away from feelings of despair and loneliness, and to promote spiritual awareness, understanding, and wholeness.

Signs and Symptoms of Spiritual Pain

When people recognize that their days in this life may be numbered in weeks and months rather than in years, they will often ask questions that scare us, such as "Am I dying?" All too often, family, health professionals, friends, and neighbors quickly turn the question aside, say "Don't talk like that, you are getting better," and offer medication, food, or drink—anything to get away from that frightening and face-to-face question. Usually, when individuals realize that their questions are ignored, they stop asking them and sink into their own small world of self-imposed isolation. They are effectively denied the opportunity to talk about the issue that is most important to them.

Some people will feel that HIV/AIDS is really unfair ("Why is this happening to me? I'm a really good person; it isn't fair."). Others believe that God is punishing them for leading lifestyles that their religious beliefs have repeatedly told them are wrong. Others express feelings of betrayal by God and anger with God.

One of the things that we Westerners most fear is the possibility of losing our independence and becoming a burden. This manifests itself in feelings of unworthiness and anxiety. When the diagnosis of HIV is first heard, many people regard it as a death sentence. They can see little point in taking care of themselves and are absorbed by feelings of helplessness and hopelessness. Life may seem utterly meaningless. The past, the present, and the future appear to be wasted.

Those whose faiths have rigid rules regarding masturbation, sexuality, promiscuity, contraception, and abortion may be overwhelmed by guilt and have no one to share this with.

People often have a real fear of how the dying process will occur. Will they be alone, surrounded by technology, or at home surrounded by loved ones? Will they be in pain? They may feel they still have so much to do, and wonder who will be there for them. A pervading sense of vulnerability and loss of control undermines the individual's ability to function in any capacity.

The good news is that so many infected people, once they have recovered from the shock, numbness, and outrage of the initial diagnosis, have not only chosen to change their lifestyles but deliberately decided that their lives will not be lost in vain and that the time they have left will make a difference to others.

CONNECTING WITH OUR SPIRITUAL PATHWAY

Exploring the Past

Exploring an individual's history of religious faith, values, beliefs, and experiences is done by simply asking them to tell you about them. The thoughts and feelings that are expressed will give you strong indications of their past and present needs.

Listeners must be sensitive to and tolerant of clients' beliefs and abstain from proselytizing their own faith and value systems. Your client may be consumed with guilt. This is perhaps the most harmful of feelings as it is consuming, inhibiting, and destructive. Indeed, a mother who has infected her unborn child may find it very difficult to not feel guilty. Nevertheless, she did not intend to become infected, and she certainly did not intentionally harm her child. Helping her to explore and validate her feelings while refusing to let her judge herself as guilty will help her change her perception and live a more hopeful life.

Anger

It is more usual than not to have anger projected at other people. Anger "is commonly projected or displaced (onto situations, doctors, nurses, family members and God). The person may not be fully aware of the true source of the anger" (Kaye, 1992, p. 261). A priest tells his congregation, "Go ahead, be angry, God has broad shoulders. He can take it." Anger needs to be allowed out. Vent it. Some people will verbally rage, others will weep, others will break things, still others will deny it and believe that they are upset, but not angry. A therapist gives an angry client a pillow and wooden paddle with which to beat it; when the feathers fly, there is usually an emotional release of the anger. Another way is to write. Keeping a journal helps to identify the real cause of the rage and promotes guidance and healing.

Fear

The exploration of the self is inhibited by real or perceived fear. Fear almost always relates to the imagined future rather than the present reality (Kaye, 1992). Fear may be of death and its unknownness, of children being left alone, of financial ruin, of hospitalization, and so forth. Until these fears are explored, resolution cannot be made. In conversations with people about their fears, I have found that when fears are confronted and talked about they seem to find a new-found ability to take care of the things that can be taken care of and an acceptance that there are some things that are beyond their power and cannot be controlled.

Forgiveness

Many of us have done things to others that we wish we had not, or we have had people do things to us that we resent, nurture, and harbor, sometimes for years. Somehow it never seems the right time to say that we are sorry or to forgive our enemy. Apologizing and forgiving can be accomplished any day, at any time, and seem to be two of the hardest things for us to do.

Ask clients if they have someone they would like to say they are sorry to, or to forgive. Encourage them to make a list of these people and to identify the action or actions that caused the harm. On the list, *we must include ourselves, for in truth, who have we injured more than ourselves. Second, let us include God on our amends list, if, for no other reason than when we do harm to ourselves, then we hurt the image of God in which we were created. (Simon, 1994, p. 60)*

Before apologizing to everyone on the list, it is important to decide whether more harm will be done by actually apologizing to an individual; will it cause more pain or is this is an opportunity to choose to change one's own life pattern so that such hurtful behaviors will not reoccur, without involving the other person?

Most will find that it is easier to contact some people than it is others. Somehow, once the process is started, the more challenging tasks become easier. One can write, telephone, or, best, go to see the person. No one has to grovel! Often one finds that the other person also wants to find reconciliation and resolution and may have some guilty feelings that need to be released. When people are able to release their past and reduce or resolve their fears, guilt, and anger, they give themselves the ability to live their lives with feelings of peace and hope.

SPIRITUAL FULFILLMENT

The pathways leading to spiritual fulfillment are diverse and numerous. What works for one is ineffective for another. There will always be those days when waking up seems an enormous effort, and our attitude is "Oh God, morning" when an obviously better start is "Good morning, God"—a cliche, perhaps, but the way in which we start our day frequently programs the rest of that day. Two of the ways that may help to keep us centered are affirmative prayer and meditation.

Affirmative Prayer

Many of us were taught our first affirmative prayer when we were very young. It is that age-old and comforting prayer that begins "Our Father, which art in heaven, hallowed be thy name." Here, with faith, the presence of God is praised. That same prayer unifies people of many languages and differing religious values and beliefs.

Although most of us no longer perceive God as a bearded ancient man sitting on a large throne, traveling through the heavens, those who believe in their own spirituality certainly do believe in some kind of powerful internal or external presence, which some call God or Supreme Being. Accessing that presence is one of the easiest things that we can do. To make affirmative prayer effective, Ernest Holmes (1927) suggested that "when you pray, go into a closet [go into your own mind] shut the door [shut out objective struggle] and the Father who seest in secret will reward you openly" (p. 146).

Some people set a time of day to pray; others pray intermittently throughout the day. Going into one's own mind at more than a superficial level requires solitude, intention, and concentrated time. Affirmative prayer does not bargain. There is no "Dear God, I promise if you get me out of this mess I'll never get into one like it again." Affirmative prayer acknowledges the presence and power of a particular supreme being, while consciously emptying the mind of fear and doubt; specifically identifies the present need (do this out loud); recognizes that the need is met through this Power; and releases the need to its greater good. When affirmative prayer is consciously practiced every day, it is truly remarkable how small and large challenges miraculously either disappear or change their form into a more manageable experience. Friendships, relationships, money, better health, and good medical intervention become unexpectedly available. For example, years ago, using affirmative prayer I described in some detail the partner that I wanted and then left it to God. Several months later we met. We knew immediately that we were meant for each other and have spent the past 17 years together. Yes, miracles do happen! End the prayer with a personal thank-you list that includes anyone or anything that touches the heart: people, animals, flowers, food, coworkers, books, boats, birds, weather, children, and grandchildren. If one of these is causing distress, visualize them bathed in a glowing white light and attempt to see them as another manifestation of God, surrounded by their own purity, although they are driving you crazy at this particular time. You will be amazed what a difference this makes to one's own behaviors and attitudes toward that person. Affirmative prayer may not improve one's physical condition, but when there is emotional healing it is almost certain to make the body feel better. After the prayer, use the next few minutes for meditation.

Meditation

Those of us who meditate find and use what works for us. I believe in having some help and use a monthly booklet published by Science of Mind. It contains daily guides to richer living written by different people whose subject matter has an uncanny way of fulfilling the need of the moment. There is a wonderful book called *The Color of Light* (Tilleraas, 1988). It contains daily meditations for all of those who are infected or affected by HIV/AIDS. The pages bring love, wisdom, comfort, creativity, validity, and growth.

How you meditate is uniquely your decision. Deliberately choose a quiet time in a quiet place and allow yourself to reach deeper and deeper inside yourself. Be conscious of your breathing, breathe slowly, and relax as much as possible. When meditation is practiced regularly, there is usually a revelation of feelings that you never knew existed. The rest of the world can be shut out until one is ready to return to it.

One recent craze has been the three-dimensional picture. To see the three-dimensional illusion, it is suggested that an easy way "is to hold the book against your nose and very, very slowly pull the book away from your face. Do not focus on the image: let the images come into focus" (Thing Enterprises, N. E., 1994, p. 4). Meditation is somewhat similar. After reading the daily page, close your eyes, let the words blur in your mind, lose focus, and allow any hidden thoughts to surface. It's truly amazing when we discover what is stored in the recesses of our minds and the closets of our hearts.

Visualization

Again, there are many different techniques, but the basic intention is the same and that is to use the "imagination to create what you want in your life" (Gawain, 1982, p. 2). Visualization is not intended to control anyone else, but to help one to focus on real or perceived needs and to assist us toward balance and self-actualization. Some people are natural visualizers. When they close their eyes and allow themselves to relax, they can "see" a picture image of what it is that they believe they need for a better, more harmonious life. Other people may not see images but will have feelings or thoughts instead. If there is discord, lack, anger, hate, fear, anxiety, or guilt present in one's life, one's spiritual being is incomplete. When visualizing, identify what is causing distress and see what needs to be done to remove it. Then visualize that whatever "it" is is already resolved. Tell this to yourself aloud and focus strongly on a positive outcome. Visualization can be used for life-limiting issues and for providing relaxation, for example, in the middle of a hectic day when taking a mental 5 minutes can transport you to a warm, golden beach or a snow-covered mountain, breathing the air, releasing the fatigue, and returning to the world that you just left restored and refreshed.

Hope

Hope is surely the most indomitable and necessary of human feelings. Without hope, life has little meaning. History has repeatedly told us of events where people, deprived of practically everything, have survived because they hoped. There are few of us who have not at some time in our lives felt deprived of hope, but the vast majority of us will find our way through the chaos and become hopeful again. Hope and our spiritual values are frequently intertwined.

When we stereotype people living with HIV/AIDS as victims, we are subliminally suggesting that they are helpless. This is not true. It seems as though infected persons who determinedly live their lives hopefully are those who live well longer. Although hope may not cure the disease, the longer people live, the better the chance that they will be alive when a cure is found. We do a disservice to anyone who is coping with a terminal illness when we label them as victims.

I am in no way suggesting that the health professional or caregiver should deny that death may occur before a normally anticipated life span is completed. I am suggesting that when hope is present, the affected individual and surrounding family members have the opportunity to live more creatively and completely, resolve unfinished business, create memories, develop a spiritual pathway, modify the "if-onlys," become involved in the community, and generally live for the day. HIV/AIDS has acted as a catalyst for many, many infected and affected people. When nobody else cared, they empowered themselves to provide care, change laws, fund research, advocate for better care and treatment, write newsletters, develop educational programs, and take the message of HIV/AIDS to schools and university systems. Without courage and hope, they could not have done all of these things.

When the disease progresses and there is a realization that death is nearing, hope can still be maintained by helping the person to "retain control, dignity and self esteem" (Rando, 1984, p. 270).

Managing pain and symptoms, visiting with family and friends, encouraging them to feel that their life here is completed, and, if they so desire, visiting with their clergy all help to comfort. If rites and rituals are valued, these should be practiced. Those who believe in a life afterwards will often say that their transition from this life to the next is appropriate and timely. A close friend is dying as this book is being written. He has repeatedly said to his friends, "I'm ready to go to my home. I know that God has a wonderful apartment waiting for me." He is a person with sturdy religious and spiritual beliefs, has made the very most of every day since he knew that he was HIV positive, and is now ready to move on.

CONCLUSION

Spirituality is not quite the same as religious beliefs. Spirituality is that roller coaster path that develops for some of us as we choose to search for the meaning of life and an extra dimension within or beyond ourselves. Our spirituality is unique to each one of us. Its individual meaning develops from our own values and beliefs that may change radically as we move toward maturity.

Spirituality is enhanced when fear, anger, guilt, and despair are resolved. Forgiving provides us with the opportunity to change those behaviors that hurt others and therefore ourselves. Affirmative prayer, meditation, and visualization can guide us to finding paths that lead to love, peace, joy, and fulfillment.

REFERENCES

Amos, W. E. (1988). *When AIDS comes to church*. Philadelphia, PA: Westminster Press.

Gawain, S. (1982). *Creative visualization*. New York: Bantam.

Holmes, E. (1938). *The science of mind*. New York: Dodd, Mead, & Company.

Kaye, P. (1992). *Symptom control in hospice and palliative care*. Essex, CT: Hospice Education Institute.

Rando, T. A. (1984). *Grief, dying and death*. Champaign, IL: Research Press.

Simon, N. (1994). *Pathways through the steps: A spiritual approach to the twelve steps of recovery*. Unpublished manuscript.

South, K. (Ed.). (1994, August). *Inter-Action Newsletter*. Washington, DC: Dean Group.

N. E. Thing Enterprises. (1994). *Magic eye III*. Kansas City, MO: Andrews and McMeel.

Tilleraas, P. (1988). *The color of light*. Center City, MN: Hazelden.

8

Dying and Death:
Challenge and Opportunity

Don't be dismayed at goodbyes. A farewell is necessary before you can meet again. And meeting again, after moments or lifetimes, is certain for those who are friends.
—Richard Bach, *Illusions*

The predominant reason that so much fear is attached to AIDS is because it is perceived as a death sentence. The previous chapters have shown that this is not necessarily true and that an HIV-positive status certainly does not mean that life is over. However, deaths worldwide from AIDS continue to grow and, until a cure and preventive vaccine are discovered, will continue to do so into the foreseeable future.

This chapter provides an overview of those issues that surround the remaining days of life; it recognizes the importance of rites and rituals, identifies the feelings and behaviors of grief, explains the phases and tasks of normal mourning, discusses the skills that are needed to listen effectively, and describes bereavement groups that are specifically designed for those who have lost a loved one from AIDS.

Bereavement should be seen as an opportunity to provide and receive care that can prevent the development of maladaptive behaviors at a later date when grief issues remain unresolved. Frequently after death has occurred, people ask why no one told them what to expect as death approached. They have expressed feelings of fear, anxiety, helplessness, despair, and frustration toward the dying person, health professionals, and other friends and family members. They say helplessly, "If only I had known what to expect I could have done this better." Being prepared helps to resolve anxiety before death and encourages a healthier, normal bereavement recovery.

Being prepared provides an opportunity for a potentially frightening experience to become one of love, beauty, compassion, and giving that is unique in its power and not comparable to any other circumstance.

APPROACHING DEATH, BEING PREPARED

The disease process from an HIV+ status into signs and symptoms, followed by an opportunistic infection, then possible multiple illnesses and an eventual terminal stage is frequently lengthy and convoluted. Unlike most other diseases, it has no established path. Over a period of years, it can have intermingling patterns of illness, crises, and wellness plateaus. This often causes infected and affected persons to develop an internal system of denial and expectation—the denial that death may and could occur and the expectation that this is just one more episode of illness from which recovery is certain. Denial is not necessarily unhealthy. It may be the only way that some people can cope. It may be used because there are so many overwhelming life events occurring simultaneously that total reality may completely destroy the ability to function. Health professionals need to be very careful before they destroy denial that they have something else to offer in its place.

Nevertheless, if increasing symptoms of fatigue, more opportunistic infections, declining cognitive function, and difficulty with interpersonal relationships become increasingly common and plateaus of wellness less common, denial, expectation, and reality will change in their impact and meaning.

Now is the time that questions such as "Am I dying?" "Does my chart say I'm terminal?" "Do you think there is life after death?" "What's heaven like?" "Will I be alone when I die?" often surface in conversation. This may be the only time that people do ask, and if there is no response they may never ask again. This indeed is the window of opportunity—use it! Frequently, the caregiver, in denial and afraid, may try to close the window by saying, "Now, you know you had a good day yesterday," "If you don't eat you won't get better," "The doctor said you're doing very well," and "How can I live if you leave me?" When this happens, it is appropriate for the counselor to ask the client if he or she would like to speak with you alone to explore these issues and gently ask that the caregiver leave the room for a little while. If the caregiver refuses to leave, which can happen, ask the client if it is all right if the questions are discussed together. Usually the client will say yes. If the client says no, then suggest to the caregiver that both of them will have the opportunity to talk about their feelings, and that it is the client's choice and desire to have a one-on-one conversation at this time. The caregiver may still refuse to leave, and the opportunity is lost. A positive outcome very much depends on the level of trust that exists between each person.

Questions such as "Am I dying?" provide an extraordinary opportunity for an open dialogue that can expose and reduce fears, reveal unfinished business, and bring a level of comfort and peace that enhances the days and hours before death. Responses should be framed in open-ended questions such as "What would that mean to you?" "Is it scary to you?" "Do you have things that you need or would like to do?" and "Do you have relatives or friends whom you would like to see?" This form of conversation can bear incredibly rewarding results. The first time I was asked the "Am I dying?" question was by a terminally ill 34-year-old woman late one Sunday evening in an acute care hospital. She was on enormous doses of opioids that were not managing her pain. She described her pain as being "as if dry ice was poured through every bone in my body." Sitting on the edge of her bed holding her hand, I asked her what would she do if she knew that she was terminally ill. She said that she would want to be discharged from the hospital, return to her own home, and embroider altar cloths and prayer cushions for her church. After a long talk, I gently told her that she was indeed terminal. She thanked me, and I left not knowing what the outcome would be. The next morning, the woman was sitting up in bed eating breakfast and was cheerful, welcoming, and rested after her best night's sleep in weeks. The amount of opioids that she was taking dropped dramatically over the next few days. She was discharged, went home, was nurtured by her family and congregation, embroidered exquisite altar cloths and prayer cushions for her beloved church and, at her death 2 years later, knew that she had completed this life's work. She needed honesty about what was happening to her so that she could make her own choices.

Knowledge is a remarkable weapon against fear. Understanding the physical signs and symptoms and the emotional process of dying helps us to see death as a normal and natural event, not as alien and frightening but as a shared time of love that cannot be duplicated.

HIV Frontline newsletter (McKusick, 1993) and the Hospice of North Central Florida have both written articles regarding approaching death. Some of their materials are gratefully used in the following paragraphs.

PHYSICAL SIGNS AND SYMPTOMS OF APPROACHING DEATH

Circulation

There is a decreasing blood supply to the arms and legs. Limbs may change to a darker color and a more mottled appearance. There is an increasing coolness to the touch.

Action. Keep the person warm with blankets. Avoid using electric blankets.

Sleeping

There is often an increased amount of sleeping, restlessness particularly at night, difficulty in rousing from sleep, and confusion on waking.

Action. Be there as much as possible, particularly at night. Turn the patient gently from side to side every 4 hours. If there is confusion, talk with the patient in a normal tone and mention who you are and what day and time it is. Never assume that you are not understood or that the person cannot feel or hear. Hearing and touch are believed to be the last of the senses to be lost.

Secretions

Oral mucous may increase and settle in the back of the throat, causing a sound called the death rattle. It occurs when the client can no longer swallow or cough effectively.

Action. Discourage suctioning; it may increase the secretions. Gently turning the head to one side may be sufficient to drain the secretions. Using a cool mist humidifier may loosen the secretions. Reassure the family and caregiver that this is normal. Prevent dryness of the mouth by applying petroleum jelly or a moisturizer. Gently swab the mouth with a nonastringent solution of bicarbonate of soda and warm water. Ask the physician for a prescription for a transdermal scopolamine patch, which will reduce the secretions.

Respiration

As the blood circulation decreases, there may be irregular respirations that may be shallow, rapid, and panting or periods of 5–30 seconds where there is no breathing. This is called Cheyne-Stokes breathing.

Action. If there is an electrical hospital bed, elevate the head of the bed to a position that will help relieve the breathing. Use pillows if an electrical bed is not available. Do reassure the caregiver and family that the breathing is not unusual, as "Cheyne-Stoking" can be a frightening experience for the untrained observer.

Incontinence

Loss of control of the bladder and bowels are caused by muscles slowly relaxing. There will usually be a decrease of urinary output. As urine becomes more concentrated, it becomes tea-colored.

Action. A catheter inserted into the bladder will prevent the involuntary flow of urine, which increases the level of comfort for the patient. Bowel incontinence should be treated by using small, moist disposable towelettes to keep the area clean, a waterproof sheet to protect the mattress, and a good supply of disposable pads to keep the patient dry and odor free.

Metabolism

The body's metabolism slows. This often causes a decreasing need for food and fluids and an increase of restlessness and confusion, particularly during the nighttime hours.

Action. Food and fluid intakes are frequently a major challenge! A caregiver's belief system, ethnic and cultural values, or perceived duty often becomes fixated on forcing food and fluids into an unwilling mouth. "If you don't eat, you will die" is a beseeching plea frequently heard. Guilt trips are forced on patients to manipulate them into eating; these come from equal quantities of love and fear, are completely understandable, and are totally inappropriate. Explain gently what is occurring: that the person is dying and to force food will only cause discomfort. Reassure them that dehydration does not cause pain and suffering. Small amounts of fluid may be given with a syringe, a rolled moist washcloth can be placed in the corner of the mouth, or, if the patient is able to swallow, very small quantities of food can be given when the patient requests. Families, friends, and caregivers may need to be guided into other ways to care, such as gentle foot and elbow massages, cool compresses on the forehead, sitting at the bedside holding a hand, playing favorite music, or reading from a familiar book of stories or poems.

Physical Pain

Too often, people who are dying are not treated aggressively for their pain. When someone moans and grimaces when turning in the bed, transferred from the bed, or firmly touched, that person is in pain whether he or she is conscious or unconscious.

Action. Pain management should continue with the administration of around-the-clock medication and increasing the type and amount of medication whenever necessary. No one should have to die in pain, whether they are infants, children, or adults. Persistent advocacy may be needed with the physician and nurse to establish and maintain good pain management.

THE EMOTIONAL, SPIRITUAL, AND MENTAL SIGNS AND SYMPTOMS

Fear

The fears most commonly expressed by patients are of the actual death event; what happens afterward, if anything; dread of going to hell and damnation; dread of burial in a dark place; fear of being buried alive; anxiety that they will die alone; and the coping abilities of their nearest and dearest when they have gone.

Action. Develop a roster of people to be with patients 24 hours a day so that they will not be alone at the time of death. Encourage patients to choose the people, as not everyone is suitable for this most intimate of life's experiences. Reassure them that their pain regimen will continue to be well managed. Explore their afterlife beliefs with them and value and respect those beliefs. Ask them how they would like the disposal of their body to occur. Cremation, burial, or vaults are options to be considered. If the decision is made before death, individuals have an increased sense of control and it will mean a lot less emotional grief for the survivors. Reassure patients that those who remain behind will be able to cope and will receive support and help.

Predeath Reality Response

I could think of no other way to phrase this. Time and again, survivors have mentioned that in the days or hours immediately before death dying persons have a period of profound lucidity when they eat well, talk with purpose and meaning, make their farewells, move into a serene place of acceptance, and appear to be poised to "let go and move on."

Action. Make the most of every precious moment. Kiss, hug, cry, hold, say whatever you most need to say, and ask pertinent questions if answers are needed.

Withdrawal and Decreased Socialization

It is normal as physical and mental mobility decrease to wish to spend this precious time with only a few people or just one person. Visitors, however well meaning and loved, mean an expenditure of energy that is becoming more and more limited.

Action. Affirm, reassure, and attempt to fulfill any requests that are made. Release the person from this life by giving him or her permission to die. Often the permission is given with ambivalence—"It's OK for you to die, but I will look after you for the rest of your life if you live." Permission given without strings is a beautiful gift of unconditional love. The survivor who is not a part of this inner circle should not feel rejected. Their place and relationship in the person's life was important, but changing needs are now being met.

Spiritual Pain

The dying and death literature rarely discuss the spiritual anguish and pain of many terminally ill people, but more and more caregivers recognize that it is often an unspoken but intense need. Spiritual pain may be expressed through feelings and expressions of depression, loneliness, unworthiness, guilt, unfairness, punishment, confusion, abandonment, isolation, and meaninglessness.

Action. If there is a specific religious denomination, ask if there is a clergyperson whom they would like to visit them or if they would like to be visited by anyone from that denomination. If there is no clergyperson available or there is no strong religious belief system, encourage patients to explore their life. This reinforces their self-esteem by recognizing that indeed they have accomplished, they are worthwhile, they will be missed, and their life does have meaning. Memories can be jogged by looking at photograph albums, listening to favorite music, recalling historical events over the past decades, and even remembering fashion styles of previous years. Reminiscence therapy, as it is called, is a marvelous way to interact as it is enjoyable, relaxing, laugh-provoking, and ultimately a way of pursuing the deepest meaning of the self.

A man who was dying in a hospital bed had an unaccomplished desire to have spent a winter in a log cabin. The imagined cabin was in a mountainous forest and was complete with snow, big dog, and large fire. He spent many happy moments "seeing" the cabin, its location, the warmth of the fire, and the peace and contentment that it brought. His mother discovered a painting that he had created years before of his dream cabin. It was brought into the hospital and hung where he could see it on the wall at the end of his bed. As he approached death, he found extraordinary comfort and spiritual harmony as he continued to explore the building, development, furnishing, and meaning of the cabin. He died peacefully, and his painting was buried with him in the family plot.

The Moment of Death

There will be that moment when breathing has stopped; there is no heartbeat, pulse, or verbal response; the jaw and mouth are slightly relaxed; and the eyes may be open, fixed, and staring. A young male laboratory technician was dying in the hospital in which we both worked. He asked me to read "The Lord is my shepherd . . ." from his Bible. As I held his hand and quietly read the beautiful words, the hand I held relaxed, and he died quietly in calm and gentle serenity.

Death is usually not nearly as scary as it is believed to be and can be a time of exquisite comfort to the caregiver.

Action. The health professional should encourage family and friends to take as much time as they wish until they feel that they have said their goodbyes and can release the body to the funeral home. If the death occurred at home and a hospice program is being used, notify them. Usually a nurse will come to the home, pronounce the death, and notify the physician and funeral home. If the person was not a hospice patient, call 911 and usually the police and emergency rescue personnel will respond. The health professional should be aware that there may be an attempt to resuscitate the person, depending on individual state laws, the interpretation of those laws by the responding emergency personnel, and whether there is a state-authorized form signed by a physician stating that the patient should not be resuscitated. If the death is in an hospital or nursing home and the family is notified by telephone, try not to let them drive to the institution alone. Someone else should do the driving. On arrival, family and friends should be allowed to spend as much time as is needed in the room with the body.

At the time of death, however prepared one believes one is and however much one wanted to see the end to suffering, there is almost always a sense of bewilderment, shock, and denial. "If only I could take back that last second so that they were still alive" is often felt and said. This is a time of confusion, diminished concentration, sorrow, depression, and distress. Children should also be prepared for the death of a close relative, as this will be a major occurrence in their lives.

CHILDREN AND DYING

Conflicts in families may arise when there are children in the home and the death of a close relative is near. In this latter part of the 20th century, the middle and upper classes of Western society have attempted to protect their children from all potential harm and perceived distress. Research psychiatrists in future years will no doubt find that this did not work to the children's advantage, but rather developed ineffective coping abilities, distorted thinking, and unrealistic lifetime expectations. With support, preparation, and comfortable, honest communication, children can participate in the dying process and will have fewer emotional problems at a later date. Children who lose a parent or siblings will have many ongoing emotional challenges. In no way should these challenges be underestimated, but the child's presence and participation will preclude some of the guilt and anger that so often is carried into adulthood by children who are banished physically and emotionally from this most loved person in their lives.

In a dying and death class, an older woman expressed her rage because when her mother died when she was 3, an aunt had taken her to an ice cream parlor before and during the funeral and on to an amusement park. When she came home, every photograph and memento and the clothes belonging to her mother had disappeared. Her father never allowed the children to discuss their mother. Years later, their grief was alive and hurting. The buried anger toward their father was enormous, but they still felt totally impotent to confront him with their individual and shared issues.

Children should be encouraged to participate in family discussions, help with some of the care, speak with and touch the dying person, and be allowed to show their emotions. They do not need to be brave for anyone, nor should they be isolated.

The first 24 hours after a death are extraordinarily busy, with funeral arrangements to be made, friends and relatives to be notified, and incoming telephone calls to be answered. This is all happening to the survivor who usually has not emotionally realized that the death is real. Arrangements made before the death help to preclude the financial and mental regrets that may follow decisions made in haste, under pressure, and at a time of sorrow and distress.

THE IMPORTANCE OF RITES AND RITUALS

The majority of AIDS-related deaths are among young people, which reverses what is perceived as the natural order of things. Whatever their age, young people are supposed to die after their grandparents and parents, not before. They are supposed to be the people of the future, not of the past. The order of beliefs is changed. That same youthful population will often have very definite ideas as to what they see as "good" deaths and appropriate funerals. A bright, vivacious 17-year-old said that she wanted "to die in a bubble bath in Paris drinking champagne." She did not die in Paris, but she had a bubble bath with a lot of laughter 2 days before her death. A magnum of champagne, which she asked be opened immediately after her death, graced her bedside table. With tears of sorrow and joy, she was toasted into her next life exactly as she had wished.

A middle-aged couple who wanted to do "everything right" asked for help to sort out the arrangements that should be made regarding the wife's impending death. She was wonderfully organized and dumbfounded her husband when she pulled out a large address book and explained to her spouse that those with red dots next to their names were those who should be notified of her death; those with green dots were those who received Christmas cards.

Not everyone can or will discuss their own funeral as it is too painful and emotionally hazardous; for those who can, however, listen carefully and either ask them to write down their wishes or record them yourself. Be sure that they are not included with the will, which is usually read after the funeral. Their religion may dictate when and how disposal of the body should occur. They may wish to choose the clothes to wear, the form of service, the person who will lead the service, and the people to participate in the service. They may wish to write their own obituary and eulogy, compose a poem, and specify the music to be played and whether there should be flowers, a donation to their favorite charity, or both. A close friend left a fat check in the envelope containing his living will, sending his friends his love and inviting his nearest and dearest to have drinks and dinner at his favorite watering hole. An empty chair was at the head of the table in his memory, and he was honored and memorialized in a way that was totally appropriate for him.

Another time, over after-dinner liqueurs, a friend's ashes, contained in a beautiful blue and gold carved urn, were placed in the middle of the dining room table. Memories of the deceased were shared in the warmth of a South Florida night with a huge full moon sailing overhead. He would have loved it!

A funeral director will be only too willing to discuss the different options for the disposal of one's body and the costs attached to the different forms of disposal. Costs can mount up extraordinarily quickly. Planning before the death can mean the difference between a rite and a ritual that reflects the life of the person being ritualized or an expensive spectacle that may or may not be representative of the person.

Funerals and memorial services should represent persons who have died as much as possible. If their desires are written down and conveyed to everyone involved in making these most sensitive of decisions and arrangements, it not only makes it easier for the survivors but avoids family conflict and relieves anxiety.

THE ROLE OF THE FUNERAL DIRECTOR

The book titled *A Manual of Death Education and Simple Burial* (Morgan, 1984) was helpful in writing the following paragraphs.

Funeral directors, contrary to popular belief, are usually remarkably helpful. They will assist with the planning before death and provide support and a variety of services after death. They provide information regarding choices in the disposition of the body so that informed decisions are made.

THE OPTIONS FOR BODY DISPOSITION

Donating the Body to a Medical School

The body is removed immediately to the designated medical school. Arrangements must be made with the intended school before death as medical schools have certain criteria and requirements. These can be ascertained by speaking with the anatomy department of the school.

Transportation may be through a funeral home, ambulance, or the school's own transportation system. The school will explain the procedure and may or may not pay for the transportation. A memorial service can be held at a later date.

Cremation

Cremation simply means the act of burning a body until it becomes ashes. In northern European countries, as demand for land has increased there is less land for cemeteries, and cremation has become more and more common. In India, the Hindu custom of burning the dead is ancient and holy. Cremation can include a viewing and a funeral service. The ashes can be scattered in a favorite place or kept in an urn placed in a niche in a cemetery or buried in the ground under a bronze tablet. One or two urns can be buried in this way. If scattering is desired, do make certain that state law allows this before making these arrangements.

Some religions oppose cremation, including the Greek Orthodox Church and Conservative and Orthodox Jews. Roman Catholics may now request permission from their bishop, and such requests are usually granted.

Direct Cremation

Direct cremation is economical because a simple wooden or corrugated container is used and there is no public viewing or funeral service. The body is immediately removed and cremated. Arrangements for direct cremation can be made through many funeral homes or direct disposition services. Disposition of the ashes may be through the disposition service or whatever method the survivor would like. A memorial service can be held at a later date.

Burial

Burial is the committal of the body in a casket into the earth, which has been prepared with some form of grave liner, usually made of concrete. Before the burial, there may be a private and public viewing for family and friends, with the casket open or closed. Whether the casket is open or closed is determined by the wishes of the deceased or the desire of the survivors and reflects their cultural or religious beliefs.

The viewing is usually followed by a funeral service the same or next day, either at a place of worship or a funeral chapel, and the casket is then removed to the cemetery. There may be a commitment service at the grave side facilitated by a clergyperson or funeral director. A huge bouquet of red carnations was at the commitment service of a Greek friend. We were invited to process past the casket, which gave each person the opportunity to say a personal goodbye as he or she gently placed a carnation on the polished wood.

Indigent Burial

If a caregiver or family has no money to pay for any form of disposition, the county medical examiner's office should be able to finance a simple burial or cremation. The office personnel will need to verify that there are no funds and will then contact a preauthorized funeral home to transport the body and to provide one or other form of disposition.

Markers

Many burials are now in memorial parks or privately owned cemeteries, which usually have clearly defined rules for bronze markers pertaining to size, number of words, placement, and maintenance. Different areas of the country, religious faiths, cultural customs, and family plots may memorialize their beloved by erecting a granite marker headstone carved and worded in a way that reflects the individual's life. This is a wonderful way to be remembered, but it can be very costly.

Memorial Services

A memorial service may be held immediately after cremation, weeks or months after a private burial or cremation, or when there are no identifiable remains. Me-

morial services provide an opportunity for people from distant places to attend
and to remember the individual in a positive manner. Memorial services may be
formal or wonderfully informal and held in settings reflective of the individual. A
dear friend died who passionately loved the outdoors. Her service was held in
a park with a broad river running by, squirrels chasing each other round the
trees, and wild parrots shouting from the treetops. Everyone dressed casually,
her favorite songs were sung, and prayers were said. Those who wished offered
thoughts that captured her for them. Afterwards, people who had not seen each
other for many months gathered and shared a quiet, peaceful, renewing picnic
lunch.

Memorial services focus on the life rather than the death of the individual,
fostering rehabilitation, bringing the image of the deceased into focus, and recalling what he or she did for the good years of their life so the survivors have a
strong, happy image to carry with them (Rando, 1984).

It is easy to see that after death has occurred there are many arrangements to be
made immediately and in the weeks to follow.

IMMEDIATE TASKS FOR CLOSE SURVIVORS

- Meet with the funeral director to coordinate the arrangements.
- Notify the deceased's attorney and ascertain whether specific funeral and
  disposition arrangements were made by the deceased if these are not already
  known.
- Make a list of family, friends, employers, or business associates who should
  be notified. Notify each by phone personally or by having a friend make the
  calls.
- Select the pallbearers and notify them.
- Write the obituary, which should include age, place of birth, occupation, college degrees, membership held, military service, outstanding work, and list of
  close survivors. Do make certain that the life partner is included. Obituaries can
  still be read in which this person is excluded. Give the time and place of the
  viewing and service. State if a memorial service is to be held at a later date and
  where charitable donations should be sent.
- If the deceased was living alone, notify the utility companies and newspapers.
  Tell the post office where to forward mail.
- Remember that burglars read the obituaries. Take precautions to make the home
  secure, particularly during the time of the services.
- Plan for disposition of the flowers after the services. Hospitals, hospices, nurs-
  ing homes, and residential facilities are possible recipients.
- Prepare a list of people who should be sent an acknowledgment of flowers,
  letters, donations, food, spiritual remembrances, and so forth that were received.
  This may be a printed card or a personal note.
- Prepare a list and write or send a printed card notifying those people who live
  at a distance of the death.
- Consider inviting a friend or relative to stay to support and help at this time.

IMMEDIATE TASKS FOR FRIENDS

- Arrange a roster of people to answer the door and telephone calls.
- Coordinate the supply of food and drinks during the viewing, funeral, and burial time.
- Purchase disposable eating and drinking utensils.
- Arrange child care.
- Arrange for accommodations for out-of-town visitors.
- Provide transportation.
- Be as flexible and available as possible.

SURVIVORS' TASKS DURING THE FIRST MONTH

- Obtain a minimum of 12 certified death certificates.
- Meet with the attorney to commence probate proceedings. Provide the attorney with a copy of the will, certified copies of the death certificate, and a full list of financial accounts.
- Notify insurance companies. File claims where applicable. Policies may include the following:

    life insurance

    medical, health, disability, travel, and accident insurance. If this was a travel related death, major credit cards, automobile insurances, and commercial transportation insurances may carry an accidental death and dismember-ment insurance benefit to which the beneficiary is entitled.

    government life insurance

    homeowners insurance

    tax-sheltered annuities

    fraternal and civic organizations' benefits

    employer-held group life insurance, which is often a separate part of the health insurance packet

    credit life insurance (mortgages, vehicles, personal loans)

Each insurance company will need a copy of the death certificate and a claim form signed by the beneficiary. It is worthwhile to remember that insurance policies usually pay the estate or beneficiary more promptly than any other benefit.

- Apply for the following benefits, where applicable: Social Security survivor benefits, veteran's burial and survivor benefits, pension benefits, and workmen's compensation benefits.
- Notify the accountant or tax preparer if the estate attorney is not preparing the final tax return.
- Notify the stockbroker to change ownership of joint or sole-owner stocks and to cancel any open orders arranged by the deceased.
- Notify the bank(s). It is recommended that savings and checking accounts remain active for 1–2 months following the death to clear all previous transactions. A longer period may be required while the estate is settled. Banks may

require a certified copy of the death certificate. Either close or change all jointly held accounts and correct the tax identification numbers (usually the Social Security number). The survivor has the right to continue to withdraw or transfer funds. Transfer the title of any safety deposit boxes. Transfer outstanding mortgages and personal loans. With regard to certificates of deposit, accounts that mature in a specific time period follow the same regulations as most savings and checkingaccounts.

- Notify the Department of Motor Vehicles. Transfer titles of automobiles, mobile homes, and boats registered in the name of the deceased.
- Notify all credit card companies. Apply for credit card life insurance where applicable. Cancel all individually held cards of the deceased within a reasonable time period, and either close or change the name on jointly held accounts. When notifying credit card companies, send a statement inquiring whether the account is covered by credit life insurance, a photocopy of the death certificate, the name and address of the personal representative of the deceased, the name and address of the attorney filing the estate of the deceased (if applicable), and either cut up and destroy or return all cards issued in the name of the deceased.

SOCIAL SECURITY BENEFITS

When a worker dies, survivor benefits can be paid to certain members of the worker's family. A lump sum payment may also be paid; generally this is $255.

Benefits may also be available to the following: unmarried children under 18 (or under 19 if full-time high school students); unmarried son or daughter 18 or over who was severely disabled before the age of 22 who continues to be disabled; widow or widower 60 or older; widow or widower or surviving divorced mother or father if caring for the deceased worker's child under 16 (or disabled before age 22) who is getting a benefit based on the earnings of the deceased worker; widow or widower 50 or older who becomes disabled not later than 7 years after the worker's death or within 7 years after mother's or father's benefits end and dependent parents 62 or older already receiving half their support from the deceased at the time of death.

Divorced Spouses

Benefits are payable to a surviving divorced spouse at age 60 or to a disabled surviving divorced spouse 50 years of age or older if the marriage was of 10 years duration or longer. Under certain conditions, children may be eligible for Social Security benefits based on a grandparent's earnings. Survivors can get benefits in most cases if the marriage was of at least 9 months duration. This information should be disclosed to the claims representative for survivors' benefits.

Income

The amount of the benefit will be determined by Social Security on the basis of the deceased's number of working quarters and the amount paid into Social Security. Eligible survivors may be required to provide Social Security with the following documentation: certified copy of death certificate or funeral director's proof of death, Form 721; proof of marriage; proof of surviving spouse's age; proof of surviving dependent children 18 or under; military discharge papers and W-2 forms of deceased, if he or she had worked within the last 2 years before death.

Benefits Mailed to the Deceased

Benefits received before date of death are entitled to be kept. Any benefits received for the following month after the date of death must be returned.

Benefits Direct Deposited

If monthly benefits are directly deposited into a bank account, contact the bank and file Form SF-1199, the Notification to Stop Deposit. Should the benefits be deposited following the death, notify the bank and the bank will refund the monies to the U.S. Treasury. The survivor should not spend any benefits received in the name of the deceased. Time to process benefits may vary, but benefits payable are retroactive from the month of application. The Statement of Death by the funeral director (Form 721) secures this.

Earning Capacity

Social Security benefits may be related to the survivor's earning capacity. The survivor should verify this with the local Social Security office for the current Specified Earning Amount, which is adjusted yearly. If a person is 70 or older, their earnings will not affect their monthly benefits. If they are under 65, for every $2 earned over the specified earning amount, $1 of benefits will be deducted. If they are over 65 (65–69 years), $1 will be deducted for every $3 earned over the specified earning amount.

MEDICARE BENEFITS

All outstanding medical bills received for a qualified Medicare recipient should be filed with Medicare on Form HCFA 1490S and Medicare Payment for Service to Deceased Patients on Form HCFA 1660. All claims should be filed through the providing doctor or service supplier regardless of whether there is an assignment. Inform clients to contact their state Medicare office for questions about medical claims.

This may all seem extraordinarily complicated, but Social Security telephone operators are helpful and efficient and will provide the appropriate guidance.

REAL ESTATE PROPERTIES

All real estate property titles should be transferred to the beneficiary. If applicable, the survivor should apply for a widowed person exemption and for homestead and disability exemption.

VETERANS BENEFITS

Benefits may be available to the survivors of an eligible veteran. Survivors should contact the local veterans service office, which should be of assistance. Those eligible for veterans' benefits include those who served in the merchant marine during wartime who were honorably discharged and received a disability pension. Benefits include a funeral and cemetery allowance, if honorably discharged and currently receiving a disability pension from the Veterans' Administration (VA); services, or if death occurred in a VA institution or other facility paid for by the VA; a United States flag; a grave marker memorialization (excluding installation); and dependency and indemnity compensation, which is an award paid to a widow or minor children of a veteran who died either in military service or as a result of a disability incurred in such service.

Burial benefits can be applied for up to 2 years following the death of a veteran. Monthly survivor benefits for eligible widows and dependent children should be applied for through the local Veterans Service Office. The office will request the following documentation:

1. copy of veteran's honorable discharge or DD Form #214
2. original or certified copy of marriage certificate
3. certified copy of death certificate
4. original or certified copy of birth certificate of children under 18, or older if attending school, or helpless before their 18th birthday
5. if there were previous marriages on either side, original or certified copy of the divorce decree or death certificate
6. VA claim number if one was issued
7. VA insurance policy or number
8. Social Security numbers of husband, widow, or children and original or current award letter, statement of other pensions, annuities, and so forth
9. funeral bills, paid cemetery property bills, or both

CIVIL SERVICE BENEFITS

The survivor should contact the Annuity Claims Office in Bayers, PA, or the Group Life Insurance Claims office of Federal Employees' Group Life Insurance in New York City for information.

RAILROAD RETIREMENT BENEFITS

An employee is considered insured under the program if he or she has at least 10 years service and is currently connected with the railroad at the time of retirement. Available benefits include death lump sum payment, residual lump sum payment, and annuities. Inform clients to send inquiries to the United States Railroad Retirement Board (299 East Broward Blvd., Room 405, Ft. Lauderdale, FL 33301; Tel. 305-356-7372).

The board will require from eligible persons a certified copy of the death certificate; marriage certificate; divorce decree; discharge from military service; proof of medical disability; if parents are those applying, proof that the employee is their child; and a railroad claim number.

The first postdeath month is usually an exhaustingly busy time of notification, resolution of legal issues, and bureaucracy. Days pass in a haze of paperwork, there is a sense of numbness, and the opportunity and ability to grieve are practically nonexistent. Frequently, because of the numbness and the busyness the individual gives the appearance of coping well. The reality of the loss may not be felt or verbalized for several weeks. Then, at a time when family and friends have withdrawn to their own lives and when the awareness of the permanence of separation reaches the head and the heart, the grieving begins.

CONCLUSION

Death is a normal and natural part of life; it will happen to each one of us. Dying and death become less fearful when there is an understanding of the emotional, spiritual, psychosocial, and physical needs of the patient and the familial caregivers. After the death, the survivor feels numbness and shock and simultaneously has a great many tasks to perform. The health professional can be of invaluable assistance before and after death by answering questions honestly, intervening when necessary, and providing practical guidance during the challenging days ahead.

REFERENCES

Bach, R. (1977). *Illusions.* New York: Delacorte Press.
McKusick, L. (1993, May/June). The end of life in HIV disease. *HIVFrontline, 13,* 5.
Morgan, E. (1984). *A manual of death education and simple burial.* Burnsville, NC: Celo Press.
Preparing for approaching death. (Available from the Hospice of North Central Florida, P.O. Box 15235, Gainesville, FL 32604).
Rando, T. A. (1984). *Grief, dying and death.* Champaign, IL: Research Press Company.

9

Grief and Bereavement: Loss and Hope

Give sorrow words: the grief that does not speak whispers the o'er fraught heart and bids it break. —William Shakespeare (1564–1616)

Grief is a 100% equal opportunity employer. No one is immune. Grief may be stealthy or sudden. It may be caused by the death of a loved one from a prolonged illness or it may be the result of an unexpected event such as suicide, trauma, natural disaster, or terrorist attack. It may involve one person or several. The grief caused by HIV/AIDS is compounded as families, friends, and health professionals not only experience the loss of one person but, unlike other diseases, perhaps of an entire family unit. Bereavement specialists are not immune to the feelings and process associated with loss. Counselors may have the benefit of intellectually knowing what is happening to them, but the pain and sorrow are as real for them as for anyone else.

This chapter addresses the process of grief and the factors that influence a healthy recovery. It identifies the cognitive and physical manifestations associated with loss and the phases and tasks of mourning. It suggests methods for intervention, including active listening, effective communication, helpful therapies, and HIV/AIDS-specific bereavement support groups.

Grief is a unique experience for each individual. There is not a grief cookbook with a tried and tested recipe to make it all better in a day or a week. Recovery times will differ and will be longer or shorter according to a number of interrelated factors that may include, but are not limited to, the following.

FACTORS AFFECTING GRIEF RECOVERY

The factors affecting grief recovery include the way individuals died and whether they were alone or in pain, died traumatically, were in an institution, were resuscitated against their wishes, and so forth. When untoward incidences occur, survivors may anguish over the memory of the death, flooded by self-blame and guilt and full of "if onlys" ("If only I had not gone out," "if only I had listened to their wishes," "if only I could have borne their pain myself," "If only I had told my father/mother/son/daughter that I loved him/her").

"'If onlys' are regrets that reflect unfinished business and may be based on reality or perception. [They are] anxiety provoking and may cause a griever to restlessly search for an opportunity to come closer with the deceased" (Rando, 1984, p. 50). It is important to deal with unfinished business before death because it is not possible afterward.

Keeping one's life current is one of the gifts that can be bestowed on our nearest and dearest, including sharing our love, thoughts, apologies, and wishes; the whereabouts of important papers, living wills, and wills; and keeping closets and drawers reasonably tidy. It is impossible to overstate how useful this can be to the survivor when death does occur.

Support Systems

HIV/AIDS is an illness that, unlike other terminal diseases, has frequently caused relatives and friends to distance themselves from the afflicted. After 15 years, it is still a disease that arrives with its own stigma and fear. It is still ignored in some cultures and regarded as a disease associated with nasty behaviors that don't affect "nice" people. Although these attitudes are changing in the West, they still exist and this may mean that the primary care provider is left with few outside support systems. When a diagnosis of HIV/AIDS is made, the affected individual and the care partner may choose not to tell others of the diagnosis for fear of stigma and discrimination and thus may self-isolate themselves. Prolonged illness does not allow time to maintain friendships as frequently all energies are focused on the needs of the patient, not on the needs of self, particularly when the caregiver, who may be the same age as the patient, is trying to keep his or her job to remain financially solvent.

Financial Solvency

One of the tragedies of the retrovirus, or indeed of any terminal disease in the United States, is that the caregiver may be left not only emotionally and physically devastated but financially destitute. This may be intensified in the case of partnerships not legally sanctioned either by marriage or common law if a will was not drawn up, clearly defining who is to receive what. For instance, property deeds may not be in joint ownership, which may leave an equally contributing life partner extremely vulnerable.

In a bereavement group, Bob told this sad story. He and his life partner Peter had been diagnosed as HIV+ 3 years earlier. His partner became increasingly sick, and Bob, a hairdresser, worked two jobs to pay the mortgage, put food on the table, and provide medications, companion care, and small comforts. Peter, dying, was admitted to a local hospital. Bob stayed with him until he died 48 hours later. Bob went home, distressed and miserable, to find the sheriff's department had closed his home by barricading the windows and nailing wooden slats over the doors. The house was papered with "keep out" signs.

Peter's parents, after hearing his diagnosis, had told him that it was entirely his fault because of his homosexual lifestyle and not to expect any help from them. Bob telephoned them in Michigan when he realized that their son was dying. They came to Florida unannounced, swept through the house while both men were in the hospital, taking furniture and jewelry, most of which belonged to Bob, and the car, and left. Bob, disbelieving and horrified, eventually spoke with an attorney. The house and car were in Peter's name. There was no will; therefore, in the eyes of the law, everything belonging to Peter legally belonged to his parents. Bob had to start his life again, grieving, HIV+, on financially rocky grounds, and responsible for an ailing sister. Miraculously, he did recover emotionally and almost financially, only to become ill, lose his health insurance, and die in an indigent bed in a publicly funded hospital. None of the extra grief and loss need have occurred if he and Peter had both realized the issues that needed to be resolved before death.

Health and Emotional Status of the Survivor

Anyone who nurses the dying is affected by fatigue, self-neglect, stress, anxiety over doing their best, and concurrent life events. The survivors may themselves be infected and may be the parents of children who are infected. Physical, sexual, emotional, and substance abuse could be present in the household. Providing basic survival needs may mean that their own grief is ignored. There may be a long-term history of clinical depression. Concurrent life events can profoundly affect the mourner's ability to survive, let alone to function.

Multiple Mourners

Over the past 14 years, all too many people have witnessed AIDS-related losses in their intimate circle of friends and family and have seen the ripple effect as close friends and acquaintances have died as a result of the opportunistic infections of AIDS. To find meaning in these deaths and lifetime changes is a continuing challenge to mourners and counselors.

Relationship and Roles

Was the survivor totally dependent on the other? Was the deceased the one who had the leadership within the relationship? Does the survivor have unexpressed or suppressed feelings of anger and hostility toward the deceased, such as "I never had a say in where we would live or the kind of house that we bought," or "Why has he/she left me in such a mess?" and "How could you leave me?" Was there unfinished business that now presents overwhelming difficulties in the matter of survival?

Concurrent Life Events

Concurrent life events can include divorce; permanent separation from previous support systems; loss of job; a move from one state to another or one country to another; loss of medical services; loss of health insurance; sexual, emotional, or physical abuse; language barriers; spiritual barriers; an ill partner or child; incarceration; and changes in social or financial situations.

Inability to Express Feelings

There are those who for many reasons—including gender, age, culture, ethnic background, perception of themselves, and natural coping style—are unable to express their true feelings and articulate their needs. These people bury their feelings; they are the ones who see themselves as having to be strong. To them, strength means that one does not give in to grief.

Suppressed grief will burst out sooner or later. When feelings are stifled, the pressure-cooker effect develops and eventually will explode, splattering whatever is in its path. Recovery will be longer and more convoluted.

Previous Lifetime Losses

Our accumulated lifetime griefs are not individual, separate single-story houses; if ignored, they will become multistoried warehouses of stored sorrows. Sorrows are not only actual deaths but those events that cause deep, often long, continued mental anguish. Sorrows are different for each one of us, and indeed, one person's sorrow may be another's gain. How we perceive and are taught to cope with sorrows from our early years on will mold our later ability or inability to grieve and cope.

Grief is a natural response to death. It presents itself emotionally, cognitively, physically, behaviorally, and spiritually (Worden, 1991).

GRIEF RESPONSES

Emotional Feelings

Sadness is the most common feeling of loss, which may be expressed through tears and copious crying. Anger may be visible, suppressed, or buried. Women find it particularly difficult to say that they are angry with the deceased. Friends and relatives usually do not like to hear and see anger toward the deceased. During the first 3 months after the death, health professionals may be the focus of anger: "If they had done that, this (death) would not have happened." Survivors almost always express loneliness, sometimes coupled with feelings of desertion and abandonment. Guilt is frequently expressed through if onlys: "If only I had told my mother that I loved her," "If only we hadn't fought just before he died," "If only I had not left the house to run that stupid errand." Anxiety may be expressed toward the future, particularly if the survivor is HIV-infected: "Who will look after me?" Children may be fearful and question whether the other parent will die: "Did I cause my parent's death?", "Am I going to be left alone?", "Who will look after me?"

There may be searching and yearning for the lost love, often expressed by looking for a visible sign of the person's presence; relief that the loved one is no longer suffering, accompanied by guilt that they feel this way; fear of the future; fear of a possible HIV-positive status; fear of the unknown; and fear for one's own ability to survive.

Cognitive Responses

There are very few people who, however prepared they believe they are, do not feel an instant disbelief and a desire to take back the last seconds of life when the last breath of the beloved is taken. On waking in the mornings after the death of one's nearest and dearest, it can take 15 to 20 seconds to realize that the partner is no longer there. Throughout the day, there is the expectation that the person will walk through the door at the accustomed time. People not only feel confused but sometimes believe that they are going mad. Their world has shattered into thousands of pieces, and there are strong, often unexpressed feelings that the pieces will never come back together again. Loss of concentration is almost certain to manifest itself, memory becomes impaired, simple tasks become monumental, driving becomes hazardous for the driver and the rest of his or her fellow travelers, and bewilderment and disbelief are a chaotic but normal part of the grief response.

Physical Responses

Physical responses to death are usually immediate and often demonstrated by an increased heartbeat, breathlessness, dry mouth, sweaty palms, nausea, involuntary tears, and mild to violent stomach cramps. As the postdeath days move into weeks, choking, hyperventilating, diarrhea, fainting, loss of appetite, and unaccountable aches, pains, and muscle weakness are often reported. Disturbances in sleep patterns occur. Sleep may be elusive or of short duration. There may be dreams and nightmares about the deceased. Severe and draining fatigue accompanied by an almost anorexic loss of appetite may be present. It requires enormous energy to struggle through the grief process, and what little energy the person has may already be going to meet everyday family needs.

Frequently, there is a continuous sensation of numbness, emptiness, and unreality. Other people speak but are felt to be at a distance. Necessary tasks are mechanically performed, but the individual feels remote and detached.

Grief Behaviors

Common behaviors in grieving people are absentmindedness, social withdrawal, hyperactivity, a repetitive telling of the actual death event, frequent visits to the site of burial, and keeping very busy. Photographs of the deceased may be destroyed or hidden or, conversely, the home may be awash in memorabilia. Belongings of the deceased may be gathered up and disposed of quickly. Getting rid of belongings in the first few weeks may be regretted at a later date, both as to who received them and the loss of memories that cannot be regained. Survivors are often advised by well-intentioned friends that they will feel better if they are not surrounded by daily reminders of the deceased. If this is left up to the mourner, he or she usually knows when it feels comfortable to sort out what is to be kept and what can now go.

The deceased may become idealized almost to the extent of sainthood and will be unrecognizable to friends and relatives. There are no hostile feelings expressed toward the individual, and they are described as having only positive traits. When these behaviors are short term and gradually change as grief becomes resolved, they are not harmful. If this thinking does not decrease over the months, it may be a symptom of a complicated grief reaction, and outside expert therapeutic intervention is indicated.

Talking and writing about death is an intellectual exercise until the death is near to our own heart. It is when the gut responds that the true meaning of death becomes apparent. Grief also is peculiarly our own. Each one of us will recover in our way, in our own time, and according to our lifetime coping skills, personality, support systems, the meaning and relationship of the loss, our financial well-being, our physical health, and other losses that may be happening simultaneously.

There is no one true way to grieve. The phases and tasks of mourning are merely guidelines for the counselor to assist in the identification of the process. They are not written in stone. Clients should never be labeled as being in a particular phase, and the counselor should recognize that people will move backwards as well as forwards in phases and tasks.

PHASES OF MOURNING

Phase 1: Denial and Numbness

Phase 1 is of conscious or subconscious denial. Survivors are "frequently emotionally numb and [perform] everyday tasks automatically" (Parkes, 1972, p. 110). They often appear remarkably capable and resilient, refuse offers of help, organize and accomplish the postdeath tasks, astound their family and friends with their calm ability to function, return to work the following week, and firmly believe that their grief recovery will be a matter of weeks. This is supported by their repeatedly being told such things as "how well you are doing," "you are so strong and brave," and "I don't know how you do it." The reality of the loss does not usually set in until 3–6 weeks after the death, at a time when a lot of the busy work is accomplished, relatives have returned home, and friends are relieved that the individual is doing so well and that they can now return to their own lives and leave the bereaved to get on with theirs.

Phase 2: Disorganization

This phase usually kicks in from 3 to 6 weeks after the death. Numbness, shock, and disbelief are less present. There is a dawning recognition that life has changed permanently and that the beloved is not returning. Loneliness is an unwanted and persistent companion, accompanied by feelings of fragmentation, isolation, and emptiness.

Persistently disorganized persons become more so. Piles of unopened mail can become mountains, dirty dishes swamp the sink, logical sequential thought is elusive, decision making is scattered and illogical, and physical appearance graphically mirrors the bereaved's internal upheaval. The immaculate self becomes rumpled and crumpled. Appearance is of little importance as the world that is known is now the unknown. Organized people will do equally bizarre things to maintain an appearance of order and control. For example, an attractive and meticulous female client's husband died and was buried with full military honors at Arlington National Cemetery. At the end of the ceremony, as is customary, she received the carefully folded national flag that had covered the casket. When she returned home, she placed the flag on the kitchen counter. She maintained her need for organization and tidiness by placing every piece of mail, including condolence letters, bills, and third-class and junk mail, under the flag. Months later when she came for counseling, the flag was completely unfolded and the mail was several feet high but invisible. She had preserved and validated her sense of her tidy self as her known world disintegrated around her.

Another client spent hours each day at the grave of his life partner. He cried, raged, yearned, and sought some sign that would tell him that he was heard. He was consumed with guilt, believing that in their shared lifetime he had not paid enough attention to his partner's needs, hadn't said "I love you" enough, and, what made him most guilty of all, had not carried out his partner's dying wish to not be hospitalized, intubated, or resuscitated.

A mother whose son died from AIDS threw herself into volunteering with those who were dying from the disease shortly after his death. She profoundly believed that this was her life's new mission. After her first patient died, she fell into a well of despair. She eventually recognized that this may indeed be her life's mission, but not until her grief work and process had time to heal and reconcile.

Disorganization moves along at its own inexorable pace. It will have many hiccoughs and may suddenly and unexpectedly return years later, triggered by a particular smell, a special song, the turn of a stranger's head, photographs, or travels to remembered places, or for no apparent reason at all.

Phase 3: Reorganization

Reorganization and reintegration is often so stealthy that it literally sneaks into the individual's consciousness without recognition. Generally, it seems to begin around 7 months after death and slowly strengthens. If there are other life losses in this period, a return to the initial phase of denial, shock, and disbelief is entirely possible.

Reorganization means that each day is not as consumed with thoughts of the loved one, sleep patterns are more normal, the tears and distraught feelings of loneliness are less frequent, memories of the life together are seen more realistically, and self-absorption lessens and commitment to others increases. There is a more positive anticipation of the future, an ability to begin defining goals, and joy in reestablishing friendships.

The period of reorganization usually contains the first anniversary of the death. This is frequently a time of challenge and confusion. Strong grieving emotions may resurface that are bewildering because the person thought he or she was doing so well. The feelings and behaviors can start days or weeks before the anniversary and may continue for a similar period after the date. This is normal, but nonetheless painful and distressing.

Phase 4: Reconciliation and Reintegration

Normal grief is an intricate and slow process without a "one-size-fits-all" pattern. Reconciliation to the loss and reintegration into life is its hoped-for outcome. Small signs of both of them will be seen before the first-year anniversary, but they are much more apparent in the second year.

THE FOUR TASKS OF MOURNING

It has been suggested that there are four tasks of mourning to be accomplished before complete healing occurs (Worden, 1991).

Task 1

The first task is to accept the reality of the loss. Until the loss is confronted and accepted, and until there is the emotional and intellectual recognition that this is truly a complete and irreversible separation (at least in this world), the process of grief is put on hold.

The denial of death was much more difficult in the early part of this century when it was customary for people to die in their own homes. We have institutionalized, sterilized, and technologized death to such an extent that it has become an abnormal event. The hospice movement has encouraged the return to death at home with the intimate involvement of family and friends, but many people will continue to die in hospitals and other institutions. Indeed, this may be their choice. Some of us feel safer surrounded by high-tech equipment, professional expertise, and the knowledge that advanced life-saving techniques will be used. However, this frequently separates the primary caregiver from the actual death, and the reality of the death is that much harder to assimilate.

Whenever the death happens, it is enormously important that the survivors be given as much time as they need to say their goodbyes before the removal of the body, not only for their emotional well-being but to help begin the process of reality and acceptance by seeing the physical change in the deceased.

Rituals help to establish the reality of loss.

Rituals such as funerals and memorial services validate and personalize the life of the deceased and allows the mourner a public and socially legitimized opportunity to display certain feelings about the lost loved one and act out emotions and behaviors necessary for resolving grief. Funerals begin the process of reintegrating the bereaved back into the community. (Rando, 1984, p. 183)

The rites and rituals following death require the friend and counselor to tread gently and carefully. Many of us are not conversant with traditional religious and cultural customs other than our own. It behooves us to learn as much as we can about other practices so that we can provide effective, nonjudgmental support and intervention with the funeral and religious entities if it is needed.

Task 2

The second task is to work through the pain and grief, which is indeed a challenge as our culture expects and wants mourners to make a rapid recovery and not discuss their grief. Grief can be profoundly uncomfortable to those unaffected by it. It encroaches on our own attitudes and feelings regarding death. Furthermore, it is a painful reminder of our own mortality and that death will inevitably happen to us.

All too often in AIDS-related deaths, the survivor is a younger person who may be both HIV-infected and a multiple mourner who has seen many friends die already. Societally, they are told that their mourning should not last too long. Company policy frequently assigns 3 days for bereavement or compassionate leave and an expectation that you will be in the office the next week as a fully functioning human being.

No longer do we wear the symbols of mourning that visually bespeak our sorrow, for example, black armbands, widow's weeds, or dark clothes. Today our mourning is hidden, internalized, and often disenfranchised. Is it any wonder that this is often a time of disorganization, confusion, isolation, and busyness? Any action that pushes away the grief is welcomed, encouraged by well-intentioned friends who advise you "get over it," "be grateful for the years you had together," "he/she would not want you to behave this way," "thank goodness that you have other children," "take a vacation," "the house is too big, sell it," "everything is going to be all right," and dozens of other cliches. The effect of this advice is to make people feel guilty and ashamed of their grief, thus discouraging recognition of the need to work through the pain and grief.

There are a variety of things that can help the grief process. This is often the time when self-blame and blaming others is apparent. Life may be wrapped up in regretful if onlys: "If only I were the one who died," "If only the doctor/nurse had done a better job," "If only someone had told me what to expect." The bereaved may repetitively recall the actual time of death and describe it in minute detail. There is recognition of the role that the person played in the relationship, not only in the sharing of the big things such as love, security, finances, companionship, and goals, but in the small practical ways such as changing fuses; being technologically competent; and being the "social secretary," preparer of wondrous meals, instigator of fun times, keeper of the checkbook, payer of bills, and handler of other taken-for-granted tasks that suddenly become overwhelming and frustrating to the survivor. A friend's biggest if only centered around a magnificent and complicated entertainment center. The printed instructions were long gone, his partner had always operated it, and he was without music because he felt foolish asking for help. No question is foolish if you don't know the answer. Asking for help is truly OK.

There is irrefutable evidence of the loss. The bed and chair are empty, the second table setting is no longer necessary, and the second car is a mute reminder. The counselor's role is to validate the loss by acknowledging and supporting mourners' feelings, encouraging the ventilation of their pain, and preventing them from physically harming themselves. To be able to do this requires listening attentively and sympathetically without judgment or advice.

Task 3

The third task is to adjust to the environment in which the deceased is missing. This means different things to different people and is affected by their age, ethnic and cultural background, spiritual and religious beliefs, support systems, financial ability to survive, concurrent life events, and the role and meaning of the relationship. With HIV/AIDS losses, it may mean not only the loss of a partner or spouse but the continuing losses of several or all of the members of a family. Concurrent life events therefore become complex issues with no easy solutions. It has to be accepted by the friend or counselor that good outcomes are not always possible and that one's best, however apparently inadequate, has to be enough.

A role change will have occurred, and adjusting to new roles is not easy. Role changes can involve the practical tasks of cooking, driving, balancing the checkbook, operating the washer and dryer, planting the garden, and buying the groceries, to name but a few.

In a broader fashion, survivors may have filled the roles of nurse, companion, and caregiver for months before the death so that now their life's role has drastically altered. No longer do they have to be aware of medications to be administered, physician's appointments to be kept, or baths to be given; indeed, their very purpose appears to no longer exist, and feelings of helplessness can occur.

The arresting of task III is not adapting to the loss. People work against themselves by promoting their own helplessness, by not developing the skills they need to cope, or by withdrawing from the world and not facing up to environmental requirements. (Worden, 1991, p. 16)

A positive commitment is needed to progress through Task 3. Developing new skills may seem overwhelming but is not impossible. Help for practical skills can be found from friends, support groups, college courses, technical programs in adult education, and the client's own determination. A father came to an evening bereavement support group with 18-month-old twins clutching his hands. His wife had died a few weeks earlier. Friends and relatives were moving back into their own routines. His immediate need was to master the laundry that was in a huge dirty pile in the trunk of his car. The group cheerfully trouped down to the local laundromat and gave him the ABCs of washing, drying, and folding. The result was a grateful dad, comfortable clean kids, and a satisfied support group who had an opportunity to help a fellow traveler along his particular road.

Women who are not used to taking charge may find themselves in the role of mother and father, as well as being head of the household, breadwinner, troubleshooter, and responsible for a variety of functions that were taken for granted before and that now seem overwhelming. This leaves little time to acknowledge and respond to their own grief or to acquire new skills. Practical help from the counselor could be finding a volunteer accountant to organize and track financial needs; accompanying the client to a meeting to discuss family issues with a school counselor and teacher; asking an HIV-knowledgeable attorney for advice; babysitting children; taking older children off to swim, play, watch a football game, or see a movie; or encouraging the survivor to join a parental support group. These are ways to provide a sense of security in a world turned upside down.

Task 4

This final task is to emotionally relocate the deceased and move on with life. For years, bereavement counselors have used the expression *letting go.* I believe that anyone who has truly loved does not let go and indeed should not let go, for this implies a banishment of the individual, never to be thought or spoken of again, that neither does, nor should, happen. Rather, the intent should be to "help the bereaved find an appropriate place for the dead in their emotional lives—a place that will enable them to go on living effectively in their world" (Worden, 1991, p. 17).

Clients appreciate being given a brief and simple summary of the phases and tasks of mourning that provides an understandable context that validates their feelings and establishes the understanding that this is a process that cannot and should not be rushed.

Grieving consumes enormous amounts of energy, and confronts and drains the mourner emotionally and physically. When reconciliation to the loss develops, the bereaved is able to move into a more comfortable place. Energy is now available to reintegrate into a new life, and the individual can accept the present and commit to the future by planning and goal setting.

The counselor is challenged to find interventions and therapies that will assist clients through their grief and bereavement to reconciliation and reintegration. Effective communication and active listening are essential to the process.

COMMUNICATION AND LISTENING SKILLS

Communication and listening skills go hand in hand. According to the *New World Dictionary* (1976), to communicate is to impart, share, make known, to give or exchange information, to have a sympathetic or meaningful relationship. The *Oxford Paperback Dictionary* (1988) states that to listen is to make an effort to hear something, to await alertly to hear a sound, to hear by doing this, to pay attention.

We communicate verbally and nonverbally, consciously and unconsciously, in a variety of ways. Verbal communication is in words, song, grunts, groans, chuckles, laughter, dialect, slang, jargon, sarcasm, hyperbole, and a multiplicity of languages that have sublanguages of their own with tonal ranges, phrasing, and speech patterns peculiar to their ethnic and cultural derivation.

How we communicate causes reactions and responses that may be directly opposite to our intention. For communication to be effective, it should be seen as a process that has seven steps.

Communication Process

Step 1 Thinking: what is it we wish to communicate
Step 2 Encoding: putting it into a form that is succinct, accurate, and understandable to the receiver
Step 3 Transmitting: how the message is sent, which may be by writing, verbally face to face, touching, or body language. Body language and facial expression can reverse a positive statement into a negative one.
Step 4 Receiver: the person who receives the message.
Step 5 Decoding: how the receiver interprets and understands the message
Step 6 Feedback: how the receiver interprets the message back to the sender
Step 7 Context: the setting or environment in which the communication is sent and received

Good communication occurs when one is comfortable with one's own feelings and emotions and accepts that another's are not the same as one's own or anyone else's. Effective communication requires clarity, openness, compassionate honesty, respect for different points of view, willingness to take risks, and recognition that individual values are different and that prejudice is harmful and potentially dangerous. Positive communication is the instrument for trust, growth, awareness, objectivity, positive regard, and, in a client–counselor relationship, the means for an eventual and appropriate termination of that relationship.

Communication and active listening are dependent on each other. Active listening requires a quiet, noise-free environment; plenty of facial tissues and somewhere to put used ones; freedom from interruption, with the door closed, telephones on hold, and beepers switched off; paying attention, attentive body language, eye contact if culturally appropriate, no furniture barriers, and no mind wanderings. Counselors should give undivided attention calmly and in a relaxed manner, avoid giving advice until it is asked for, and should not devalue feelings, whatever they are, but unconditionally accept whatever is expressed. There should be recognition that mourners cannot always express themselves in a coherent way (don't finish clients' sentences for them); recognition that there may be communication differences because of language, culture, upbringing, age, sex, sexual preference, and lifestyles; and feedback to clarify that you understood what was said. Nonjudgmental, focused listening is a gift beyond price that brings growth, understanding, and empowerment to the client and the listener.

Relationship Review

Often people express anguished feelings of not having done enough before the death. Reviewing these past events and behaviors with them will, more often than not, graphically show them that they did indeed do their very best according to their ability. This helps to assuage guilt that they do not need to feel in the first place.

The Libido

One of the bereavement traps is the libido, particularly if, because of the deceased's increasing illness, intimate sexual actions had not happened for a long time. Often there is the belief that a sexual relationship during bereavement will improve one's well-being, particularly as love in our society is so frequently equated with sex. Suggest friendship, support groups, cold showers, masturbation, relaxation techniques, physical exercise, and indeed anything that works, but do discourage an actual affair. More often than not, searching for comfort in another's arms results in a broken relationship accompanied by self-disgust, guilt, anger, and many steps backward in the grieving process.

Financial Loss

The loss of a partner can mean financial devastation, but if it is at all possible, do discourage any major moves to a new home, state, or country or a change of jobs until the grief has lessened and it is easier for the client to make informed decisions.

Activities

Very often the bereaved are working people and are able to keep themselves together during the weekday only to fall apart in the evenings and on weekends when they are confronted with a home of memories and aloneness. Suggest activities that will provide some companionship and require little effort such as a walk on the beach, a movie, or a delivered or takeout dinner shared with a good friend. It is not unusual to see an increase in alcohol, nicotine, or caffeine use. Usually this is temporary. Discuss this with clients; remind them that alcohol, smoking, and excessive use of prescription and nonprescription medications are habit forming and only briefly assuage the pain.

The grief process is accomplished in small steps, not in huge strides; thus, small attainable goals are more effective than large grandiose goals that are invariably doomed to failure. Agreeing to exercise two or three times a week, having a decent meal a day, allotting a daily time to mourn, and sleeping well are achievable goals that will help in their recovery.

There are three therapies that seem to have particularly helped this client population. They are taking a daily time to mourn, keeping a journal, and daily affirmations.

THERAPIES

Grief is a time when dysfunction can be considered normal. However, this dysfunction often makes the ability to struggle through each day a monumental task, made more challenging if the individual has to work to survive.

A Time for Mourning

Establishing a specific mourning time before or after work means that the individual can function fairly well during working hours. It is done by choosing a quiet place, setting the alarm for 20 or 30 minutes, and "spending time" with the deceased. Talk, laugh, cry, shout, rage, share the day, share memories, and be with the person as closely as possible. This accomplishes several things. It brings the lost love near to the heart, helps to work through the pain of grief by resolving unfinished business, acknowledges the multiple facets of the loss, recognizes that one is surviving, and prevents idealization of the partner. Most of all, it allows individuals to get through each day with some kind of coherence, knowing that later they can grieve as intensely as they need to. As the grief process unfolds, the daily time for mourning will lessen.

Keeping a Journal

Something magical happens between the head and the heart when mourners choose to grieve through writing. "The cathartic power of writing provides emotional release and can eventually help life to proceed more easily" (Rainer, 1978, p. 53). Keeping a journal purges rage, sorrow, hate, fear, despair, depression, and pain. The written words are reminders of the difficult paths that feet have stumbled along. Words provide memories and histories of a shared relationship and offer validation of the lost love's life. Writing prevents the idealization of individuals by making them real. Their habits are seen more objectively, and although many of these habits were endearing, some were annoying, irritating, and frustrating, which is an ordinary human condition. If any kind of abuse was present but denied, writing may well cause this veil to be pulled away.

When the person is perceived in all his or her facets, lovely and unlovely, future relationships will be easier as the new person will not have to replace the other or attempt to live up to this imaginary perfect, sainted person.

Affirmation

Grieving individuals frequently find it impossible to believe that life is still full of hope, beauty, challenge, opportunity, and meaning. Affirming life is definitely not on their agenda at this time. However, there are still small and large positive things happening around them.

Invite them to acknowledge these positive things by taking 5 minutes in a quiet spot to focus on and to list aloud some good events, such as letters from friends, the sunrise, a bird singing, an unexpected loving phone call, financial stability, a caring pastor, a faithful pet, or whatever is good in their lives. Concentrating on good things helps to relieve sorrow, if only temporarily; provides a measure of comfort; recognizes the beauty of ongoing life; and develops a sense of inner peace and security.

Many people will stumble through the grief process either alone or with the help of a good, nonjudgmental friend; a supportive family; empathetic coworkers; and individual bereavement counseling. Others will reach out for HIV/AIDS-specific bereavement support groups, which are now available in a number of locations throughout the country.

HIV/AIDS BEREAVEMENT GROUPS

In 1987, I was employed by a hospice program as its director of bereavement. The agency had seen a steady growth in its services to persons with AIDS since

1983 but had very little representation of the survivors from that population in the regular bereavement groups. These groups were predominantly composed of older people, mainly women, whose spouses had died from cancer, heart disease, or other terminal diseases but rarely from AIDS. It is customary at the first session of the 8-week group to ask each person to introduce him- or herself, name the person being mourned, the relationship to the group member, and the cause of death. Significantly, it was found that the few present who were grieving an AIDS-related death never gave the cause as being AIDS-related but stuck to the more societally acceptable losses such as pneumonia, leukemia, lymphoma, and unknown causes. By doing this, they seemed to limit their healing process as the ability to explore their feelings and issues was choked by their understandable fear of speaking the truth.

Thus started an HIV/AIDS-specific bereavement group that learned its own developmental lessons as it went along. It was different from the more usual bereavement support groups because the participants were generally younger and had many questions relating to grief and to HIV/AIDS, so that the educational requirement was as intense as the need for support. "The goal was to provide a safe, secure environment where individuals had an opportunity to develop trust and to discuss the reality of their loss with others whose loss was related to AIDS" (O'Donnell, 1989, p. 1).

The goal was achieved in a variety of ways and included the careful selection of facilitators, the development of content and group rules, the use of relaxation and guided imagery exercises, ongoing and updated HIV education, a lot of reminiscence therapy, continuous evaluation, and a willingness to change the content when participants' needs were not being met.

In the beginning, three facilitators ran the group. They were a physician specializing in HIV and a psychotherapist—both hospice volunteers—and myself. We shared commitment, humor, empathy, and a willingness to learn; nonconfrontational and nonjudgmental attitudes; knowledge of community resources; and an intense desire to see the group work.

Outside speakers were sometimes invited. They included an attorney, tax consultant, pastoral chaplain, Social Security representative, masseuse, physical therapist, nutritionist, and representatives from drug manufacturers involved in the medications of HIV. The use of outside speakers depended entirely on the needs and wishes of the group.

Rules for the group were developed by the group and included a heavy emphasis on confidentiality; no comparisons of deaths, as no one's death experience is less or more significant; listening to each other; only one person speaking at a time; sharing telephone numbers but not addresses; punctuality in beginning and ending; smoking at any time but only in designated areas; no drugs or alcohol on the premises; allowing persons who arrived drunk to stay if they were not obstreperous; tidying up the room before leaving; and leaving together for personal safety.

The contents of the sessions included a description and discussion of the grief process and grief work; reminiscence therapy assisted by tapes, cassettes, photographs, music, songs, and poems; recognition and resolution of anger, guilt, shame, and blame; communication and listening skills; pre- and post-HIV testing; disease process and current interventions for HIV spectrum disease; nutrition, exercise, and sleep; stress and time management; religious and spiritual issues; coping with special anniversaries and holidays; memorials; and moving on. The reminiscence therapy session became the most therapeutic. Photograph albums, tape recordings, videos, and other personal memorabilia were brought in. The sharing released many emotions and seemed to form the cohesive glue that bonded the group to each other, so this session was always held early in the overall program.

The sessions are for 8 weeks and are closed; that is, no one else can join the group after the second week. The only criteria for joining the group is that the cause of the bereavement be from an AIDS-related illness. People in the groups are parents, siblings, life partners, caregivers, friends, relatives, buddies, and health care professionals. Participants join the group from 6 weeks to 13 months after the date of death.

The group ends with a potluck supper. The food is fabulous, and nothing is quite as moving as sitting at a table with people who, 2 months before, could barely hold a conversation without tears. They have now shared and validated their sorrow and have some tools to help them heal through the following months.

Out of the groups have come quilts for the Names Project, each stitch, sequin, star, tassel, baby's rattle, and message a loving and lasting tribute to those who have died. The quilts are a little like keeping a journal, for, similar to writing, as the stitches are sewn wounds begin to heal.

The first group was diverse in age, culture, gender, belief system, profession, and ability to articulate. At the end of the 8 weeks they refused to say goodbye! There was a strong desire to give something back as a memory to those loved ones who had died and to help those who grieved. The decision was made to write a step-by-step guide to running an HIV/AIDS-specific bereavement group. Meetings were every other Tuesday evening for a year and a half. Eventually, the manual was produced in a three-ring binder format and was named *The Sheltered Heart* by one of the mothers, and the cover was designed by a young man who received the finished book 3 days before his own death. The manual received the National Hospice Organizations President's Award of Excellence for staff training and education in 1989. The plaque was received by a group member who had become an extremely active and beloved hospice volunteer and educator and to whom this book is dedicated.

Children must not be forgotten in the grief process. Nothing is more shattering to a child than the loss of a parent or a sibling, and yet their grief is often not recognized, acknowledged, or validated. Children's grief, if ignored, will almost certainly present itself again later in their lives. It will not go away on its own.

CHILDREN AND GRIEF

Children express loss differently than adults, and because they are not always in tears or visibly mourning are often believed to be managing very well when in actuality their whole world is caving in. Polumbo (1978) suggested that

1. Children do mourn, but differences in mourning are determined by both the cognitive and emotional development of the child.
2. The loss of a parent through death is obviously a trauma, but does not in and of itself necessarily lead to arrested development.

3. Children between the ages of 5 and 7 years are a particularly vulnerable group. They have developed cognitively enough to understand some of the permanent ramifications of death, but they have very little coping capacity; that is, their ego skills and social skills are insufficiently developed to enable them to defend themselves. This particular group should be singled out for special concern by the counselor.
4. It is important also to recognize that the work of mourning may not end in quite the same way for a child as it does for an adult. Mourning for a childhood loss can be revived at many points in an adult's life when it is reactivated during important life events. One of the most obvious examples is when the child reaches the age at which the parent died. When this mourning is reactivated, it does not necessarily portend pathology but is simply a further example of working through the death.
5. It is important for the mental health worker to develop preventive approaches for children who have lost parents. The same tasks of grieving that apply to the adult obviously apply to the child, but these tasks have to be understood and modified in terms of the child's cognitive, personal, social, and emotional development.

Intervention

Many children are not going to have access to bereavement counselors or support groups. However, more public school systems are developing support groups, and other facilities may be offering them. If one is not available, starting one may be necessary. To help, the Bellin Hospice Program in Green Bay, Wisconsin, has developed a Leader Manual titled *Bereavement Support Group for Children* (Haasl & Marnocha, 1990). This is a manual full of practical information that starts with developing a brochure, moves to outlining the topics for five sessions, and finishes with blank pages for the facilitator's notes. The purposes for each session are outlined, activities are described in detail, and the materials that will be needed are listed.

Chapter 7 in the manual identifies 13 common grief responses that are experienced by children. Following the description of each grief response are caregiver techniques that are extremely useful for those parents, caregivers, and guardian and foster parents who are unable to have children attend a group. Reading about children's grief will often develop understanding and help the caregiver to help and support the child. One suggestion is the excellent book *Explaining Death to Children* (Grollman, 1967).

Children who lose close family members are always at risk. The more that we understand, acknowledge, validate, and support their grief, the more possibility there is that they will learn to grieve healthily, to live with their loss, and to find inner resources and wisdom to develop their lives creatively and fully.

CONCLUSION

Bereavement and grief are a natural part of our lives. Marking the death with some form of ritual provides the living an opportunity to validate and memorialize the life of the deceased, to provide support to each other, and to begin the first task of mourning, which is to accept the reality of the loss.

The funeral may be the first time that geographically separated parents discover that their adult child has died from an AIDS-related illness. To find this out at the time of death can cause an overwhelming sense of helplessness and frustration. They may be finding out the cause of death and their child's sexual preference and meeting their child's friends for the first time in unfamiliar surroundings and, no matter what the previous relationship, will need sensitive, nonjudgmental support. Sharing memories is a powerful and supportive intervention that captures the recent history of the deceased and reduces the emotional isolation of the survivors.

Grief has its own signs, symptoms, and behaviors. Healthy grief resolution can be accomplished by understanding and following the tasks of mourning. Good communication and listening skills along with other therapies are essential for positive outcomes.

HIV/AIDS-specific bereavement groups provide an opportunity for the understanding and reconciliation of grief through an atmosphere of confidentiality, mutually shared loss, knowledge, and empathetic support.

Children have their own way of mourning and need ongoing support and understanding.

The grief process cannot be hurried but must continue at its own pace. Grief can provide an opportunity for personal identification, exploration, and growth that can positively alter the mourner's future life in ways that were undreamed of before.

REFERENCES

Grollman, E. A. (1967). Explaining death to children. Boston: Beacon Press.

Guralnik, D. (Ed.). (1976). New world dictionary of the American language (2nd ed.). Cleveland, OH: The World Publishing Co.

Haasl, B., & Marnocha, J. (1990). Bereavement support group program for children. Muncie, IN: Accelerated Development.

Hawkins, J. M. (Ed.). (1983). The Oxford Paperback Dictionary (2nd ed.). Oxford: Oxford University Press

O'Donnell, M.C. (Ed.). (1989). The sheltered heart. Ft Lauderdale, FL: Hospice Care of Broward County Inc.

Parkes, C. M. (1972). Bereavement. New York: International Universities Press.

Polombo, J. (1978). Parent loss and child bereavement. Presented at the Conference on Children and Death, University of Chicago.

Rainer, T. (1978). The new diary. Los Angeles: J.P. Tarcher.

Rando, T. A. (1984). Grief, dying and death. Champaign, IL: Research Press.

Worden, J. W. (1991). Grief counselling and grief therapy (2nd ed.). New York: Springer.

10

Managing Stress:
Recognition and Intervention

Happiness is a perception of our minds, not a reflection of our situations. On days when everything goes wrong—days full of mistakes, accidents, rejections, noise—we can still be happy. —Jennifer James, *Windows*

I became involved with the hospice movement in the mid-1970s after observing that people who died in hospitals frequently did so with little familial support, with little control over their own lives, or without any opportunity to finish their unfinished business. Their spiritual, emotional, and physical selves were rarely treated in a holistic manner, and effective pain management was practically nonexistent.

In the pursuit of developing a hospice program, it was impossible to ignore my personal values, beliefs, and behaviors. I knew intellectually that working solely with people who are dying, and with their loved ones, would be stressful. I believed that I had reasonably intact coping skills and that this new adventure would not be too arduous. Little did I realize that the daily challenges would not be just from families, but from physicians, clergypersons, social service departments, health bureaucracies, employers, employees, and most challenging of all, my own frustration with myself because I did not have all the answers; indeed, sometimes I didn't have any. I often became the rescuer instead of the counselor, and I rarely knew when to say no.

Persons infected with AIDS and their surrounding support systems need our intervention and care not only during times of crisis, but often over a long period of time. Health professionals do get involved and attached emotionally and are themselves subject to multiple feelings of loss and distress when clients die.

If any of the above sounds familiar, read on! This chapter defines stress and stressors, identifies the characteristics and behaviors that cause distress, which can lead to burnout, and suggests methods of intervention in the workplace and the home. Do remember that what paralyzes the mind for one is caviar and champagne for the other.

You may question why so much is written about organizational structures and good office management. The reason is that when a program is poorly managed it becomes a systemic stressor for its employees, often leading to high staff turnover, increased sick leave, and poor performances. A program that understands and delivers its mission and listens to and is fair to all its employees is one that is structured, dynamic, time efficient, motivational, and rewarding and leads to an enjoyable workplace.

DIFFERENTIATING BETWEEN STRESS AND STRESSORS

A few examples are as follows: Stress for me is when the alarm clock rings early in the morning, running out of time because I try to stuff too much into a nonexpandable time frame, people not being on time, always being responsible for planning meals and cooking them, and missing our mail carrier when a letter really needs to be posted that day. For me these are healthy stress situations. Without the alarm, I'd miss the beginning of the day and all the possible excitements that the day might bring. Managing this kind of stress is as easy as picking up the telephone and making a dinner reservation!

Researchers on stress have generally discussed stress versus stressors. Vachon (1987) quoted Antanovsky:

He sees stress as evolving from exposure to stressors. A routine stimulus is seen as being one to which the person can respond more or less automatically. A stressor, however, can be defined as a demand made by the internal or external environment of an organism that upsets its homeostasis, restoration of which depends on a non-automatic and not readily available energy-expending action. (p. 3)

Homeostasis is

1. the tendency to maintain, or the maintenance of, normal internal stability in an organism by coordinated responses of the organ systems that automatically compensate for environmental changes.
2. any analogous maintenance of stability or equilibrium, as within a social group (Guralnik, 1976).

If stressors are not managed and become prolonged, they may become overwhelming and lead to what is often referred to as *burnout*. Burnout is definitely not a desirable outcome.

Burnout can be insidious because we may not recognize it when it is happening to us. Feelings of emotional and physical exhaustion, occupational fatigue, cynical attitudes, and withdrawal from patients can all be attributed to outside circumstances or temporary lapses in effort. (Rando, 1984, p. 440)

"Unmanaged stressors can lead to burnout which in turn can manifest in a variety of signs and symptoms or groups of diseases including heart attacks, migraines, ulcers, colitis, diabetes, auto-immune diseases, backache, tension and arthritis" (Blattner, 1981, p. 424).

Our intent should be to understand the nature of stressors, identify our own stressors, and find individual methods of intervention to manage our stressors.

STRESSORS

Common Stressors

The majority of stressors are found in our immediate environment at home and at work, personality variables, personal value systems, lifestyles, and concurrent life events.

The Environment

Environmental stressors can be physical, psychosocial, and emotional.

Much HIV/AIDS treatment and care is delivered in the client's own home. Physical safety may well be an issue, particularly when visiting clients during the night in poorly lit unknown neighborhoods. Safety in the home itself can be a factor, for example, if clients become confrontational. Our environment may be thick with cigarette smoke, clogged by dirty air conditioning filters, extremely cold, or uncomfortably hot. It may be noisy, unnaturally quiet, hostile, or crowded with traffic. None of the above is conducive to a healthy state of mind.

Our Psychosocial and Emotional Environment

The environment at home may be one of peace or one of turmoil. At work it can be one of relative harmony or one of ambiguity, tension, conflict, crowding, insufficient resources, lack of communication, work overload, too much paperwork, too many bosses, a title without authority to make decisions, bad fits of personnel to the job, and unrealistic expectations of the organization and of self. Our external environment directly affects our personal well-being. A caring environment at home and at work can mean the difference between managing everyday stress and the eventual inability to function adequately. Conversely, an uncaring environment can lead to visible signs of burnout. Burnout may manifest itself as a lack of self-esteem and loss of concentration, which in turn can cause the loss of one's job and decreasing physical and emotional health.

Personality Variables

Personality variables that are part of our individual makeup will affect our attitude toward stress and the level of our stressors. Our motivation, expectations, and self-responsibility are closely interrelated and play major roles in the amount of stress and the type of stressors that come into our lives.

"Job stress might well develop when there is a discrepancy between the individual's motivation for seeking a particular job and the supplies for meeting that need existing within the job environment" (Vachon, 1987, p. 20). For example, individuals applied for and received appointments to new jobs in an HIV/AIDS organization to find that neither the employer or the employee had clearly identified their individual expectations before employment, job descriptions were non-existent, and resources were unavailable. The employees then had to reroute their expectations. Motivation was sometimes lost or weakened in the process. When motivation is lost, the individual will have little opportunity to develop the sense of belongingness and connectedness that Maslow (1954) defined in his hierarchy of needs.

Maslow's (1954) Hierarchy of Needs

Abraham Maslow is considered to be the father of humanistic psychology. His theory of motivation is used by many of the helping professions. He visualized his theory as a broad-based triangle; needs moved through five steps to the peak that was self-actualization. Basic needs such as air, water, food, shelter, sleep, and sex were at the base of the triangle. The other steps from the base were safety, belongingness, ego status, and growth needs. They provide an understandable highway toward one's own goals. If stressors take over the self, however, we may never make it to safety, let alone self-actualization.

Personality and You

Much is written about personality and coping styles, particularly regarding Type A and Type B personalities. Identifying one's personality type will give some clues as to probable behaviors and coping styles.

Type A personality. The Type A personality is definitely the superachiever. This type has prioritized goals, makes efficient use of time, moves up the corporate ladder, and is competitive at work and play, a workaholic, impatient with slower coworkers, often disengaged from intimate relationships, and inordinately distressed when situations are not within his or her control.

Friedman and Rosenman (1974) defined a Type A behavior pattern as

an action-emotion complex that can be observed in any person who is aggressively involved in a chronic, incessant struggle to achieve more and more in less and less time and if required to do so, against the opposing efforts of other things or other persons. (Vachon, 1987, p. 25)

They also found the "Type A personality predisposed to coronary artery disease" (Blattner, 1981, p. 159). Men are traditionally regarded as being more likely to be Type As. However, coronary artery disease is now the number-one killer of women in the United States. Whether this is direct result of more women joining the workforce or whether there is better research on women and disease remains to be seen. Type As of either sex can be challenging to work and live with.

Type B personality. Type Bs tend to be laid-back, easygoing, "time-is-no-object" individuals. Type Bs usually do not feel the need to challenge, compete, be the center of attention, hurry other people along in their conversations, or talk, eat, move, and walk rapidly. Type Bs tend to take time to smell the roses. All of the above does not mean that they will avoid stressors, but how they respond to them will be different than the Type A individual.

We are made up of a variety of personality traits that will be different in each individual. We may be introverted, extraverted, critical, creative, assertive, aggressive, intuitive, sensitive, thoughtful, indecisive, judgmental, perceptive, enthusiastic, pragmatic, aware, oblivious, analytical, theoretical, vibrant, dreary, practical, sociable, alienated, systematic, organized, messy, controlling, consensus seeking, or impossible. Most of us are made up of all sorts of personas, some of which are more dominant than others. The challenge to HIV/AIDS organizations is to learn to work with each other by understanding that each person, regardless of his or her personality, has skills and talents to bring to the organization. Successful managers can motivate teams to work productively together when they recognize, understand, and use different personality traits in tasks that are most logical and emotionally rewarding to the individual.

Personal Value and Belief Systems

Our values and beliefs develop from our culture, religion, spirituality, biological family, political system, education, self-perception, and self-awareness. These beliefs about ourselves will often dictate the kind of coping mechanisms that we develop. In the 1940s and 1950s, British children were brought up to believe at home and at school that "there is no such word as *can't*" and "if at first you don't succeed, try, try, try again." We grew up believing that our country was the most honorable and the best. It was a major challenge to my own value system to discover when moving to the island of Jamaica in the early 1950s that that was not necessarily how Jamaicans felt about my beloved country. Furthermore, they were vocal in their derision, political in their actions, and couldn't wait to welcome independence. It was at an early and impressionable age in my transition into adulthood that I realized that individual family and national values are very different. Ultimately, I passionately embraced these differences, but it took a while.

People in the helping professions can often fall prey to these personal value systems. Because we believe that our role is helping others, no burden is too much, negative feelings should not be allowed, our emotional cupboard is never bare, we are always in touch with the latest medical advances, and, of course, we will always recognize when our stressors have overtaken us. When we fail to acknowledge our stressors, it is not surprising that life becomes scarily overwhelming, effective decision making is impossible, and getting up each day becomes a major struggle.

Lifestyles

Lifetime patterns, behaviors, and thoughts affect our ability to manage stress well. Behaviors that affect us negatively include smoking, excessive alcohol consumption, overeating, always eating junk food, using illegal drugs, misuse of legal medications, little or no physical exercise, disruptive sleep patterns leading to fatigue, moving from one harmful relationship to another, forgetting or refusing to use car seatbelts, putting ourselves in life-threatening situations such as attempting to rescue a drowning person when our own swimming skills are limited or rushing into a burning building without protection or a fire extinguisher, scuba diving without a buddy, parking the car in dark, poorly lit places and leaving it unlocked, leaving home without locking the door, and never finding time for medical check-ups.

Thought patterns that are harmful to us include believing that "I'm not good enough," "I always have bad luck," "Nobody really likes me," "Other people are in charge of my destiny," "I'm not responsible for my behaviors," "I can never change," "I don't trust anyone else to look after my clients," "My plans never work out," "It's bound to rain tomorrow because it's my day off," "I don't deserve a good life," "I'm indispensable," "I know all the answers," "My way is the right way," "I'm angry all the time," "It's never my fault," "I'm scared of them because they are different," "I really want to say no but I'm afraid I'll hurt their feelings," "I can't ask for help because I'm supposed to be the strong one," "The world is violent; I'm afraid I will be hurt," and so forth. I expect the majority of people reading this book have thought some or all of these things at some time. They work against our well-being when they reflect our thoughts all the time.

Life Events

The events that happen to us in our lives can affect our environment, lifestyles, behaviors, and thoughts. My personal belief is that life events are given to us to provide invaluable opportunities to analyze and clarify our own and others' reactions and responses, to change those behaviors if they are harmful, to learn lessons so that we do not continually need to relearn them, and to use the negative events for positive outcomes. It sounds simple, but positive outcomes usually require us to recognize harmful behaviors and events and have the desire and commitment to change them. This can take a while, or it may never happen.

Certain life events are beyond our control: the death of a loved one, violent physical attacks, wars, hurricanes, floods, tornadoes, and earthquakes are some examples. Nevertheless, the better we manage our stresses, the better we are able to manage life's larger challenges.

Stressors can sneak up on us so insidiously that neither oneself, coworkers, or administrators will recognize what is occurring. To avoid this, we need to learn to identify our stressors and intervene early rather than too late.

Stages of Stress

There are three progressive stages associated with stress: The first stage is physical and emotional exhaustion and the beginning of other physical symptoms; the second stage is the development of a negative attitude toward clients, with decreased energy applied to work; and the third stage is a feeling of total disgust with work, with previous symptoms becoming extreme. By the third stage, burnout may be irreversible.

Signs and Symptoms of Overload and Burnout

Some of the signs and symptoms are frequent and unexpected crying jags, irritability, criticism, cynicism, excessive eating and drinking, seeing clients as "cases," inability to perform routine tasks, increasing paranoia, change in appearance due to a negative self-image, lack of concentration, extreme fatigue, inability to feel anything, withdrawing, isolating oneself, accident proneness, a "who cares" attitude, increased anxiety, hopelessness, frustration, anticipating the worst, difficulty in communicating, and physical illnesses.

Most people heading toward burnout exhibit only one or two of these signs and symptoms, but they are warning signals that should not be ignored. If intervention occurs early, a positive outcome should be expected. If intervention occurs late, then the results may be challenging and protracted.

INTERVENTION STRATEGIES

We as individuals need to take back personal responsibility. We alone are responsible for how we choose to live our lives. Everyone from politicians to criminals seems to blame everyone else for everything bad that happens to them. Yes, there are events that we cannot control, but there are any number of things that we can control.

Personal Responsibility

We can choose to eat sensibly, exercise moderately three to four times a week, join a "quit smoking" class, limit alcohol intake, and seek help to stop a drug habit. Boundaries can be established for children, and adults can attend a parenting class or join a support group. By saving a small amount of money each week, developing time management skills, and stopping procrastination, we can keep our lives current and learn to live within our means. Protect your health by having an annual medical checkup, visiting an optometrist when your vision begins to change, having a hearing test, taking time to grieve, getting the hepatitis B vaccination if employed in an at-risk job, and being checked annually for pulmonary tuberculosis. It is also important to take time out to relax and do things that we enjoy: spending time with our nearest and dearest; developing a hobby; playing; flying a kite; throwing a frisbee; joining a support group; writing a diary; turning off the news and turning on the music; reviewing television viewing and deliberately watching some comedies; collecting cartoons; refusing to discuss work at breaks and mealtimes; practicing forgiveness; learning another language; developing computer skills; joining a dance class; spending a day saying only upbeat things; trying meditation, relaxation, and visual imagery; and making an effort to be good to ourselves for at least 15 minutes every day.

STRESS IN THE WORKPLACE

One of the biggest areas of tension in the workplace is that which involves any form of communication. Poor communication is repeatedly listed as a major stressor. Poor communication is a downhill path leading to a lack of motivation, an increasing sense of helplessness, and an inability to deliver services skillfully and effectively.

Many HIV/AIDS grassroots organizations were begun by enthusiastic volunteers who brought their individual talents and agendas to a small group of likeminded people. Communication was often accomplished by shouting through an open door into the next office, management styles were varied, written policies were almost unknown, job descriptions were unknown, money was tight, and the thrust, rightly, was toward doing rather than toward developing organizational policies and procedures.

As the HIV epidemic spread and financial resources eventually became more available, these same agencies grew. This did not always happen easily. Agendas could no longer be individual, employment had to have structure, and long-term goals and resources had to be developed. Good communication was the key to effecting a comprehensive and positive change that could be supported by old and new employees alike. Sadly, some of the original visionaries were unable to make the change from an individual status to a much larger group, some because they themselves were infected, became ill, and died and others because they lacked the necessary business acumen and were unable to adjust to the changes required of them. Their gifts should never be forgotten—they brought advocacy, caring, political know-how, and passion that is not always as visible in some of those same agencies today.

For the good of the agency, the individual, and ultimately the client, it behooves us to understand and develop good office communication skills. This is especially important in offices dealing with HIV/AIDS. Effective communication has to start at the top. How the executive director or chief executive officer communicates affects every department within an organization, particularly those working in the HIV/AIDS community. Some of the things that promote and maintain good communication are the following.

Organizational Philosophy and Mission Statement

This should be a clear and concise written statement developed by the governing body that precisely identifies the agency's function. It should be placed at the beginning of the policy and procedures manual. It should be articulated at job interviews. All employees should know and understand its contents. As agencies grow, the mission may change. This is a natural part of growth. If the mission does change, the mission statement should be rewritten and all employees informed of this.

Job Interviews

Job interviews are time consuming, and all too often neither the employer or interviewee feels satisfied with the results. Employing the wrong person is frequently costly financially and emotionally. Probationary training periods take time, effort, and money. If the end result is letting the individual go, the hiring cycle is begun again and could have a similar outcome. This is an enormous waste and places added stressors on employees.

Reducing the Waste

Planning the job interview takes time, but clarifying the requirements and the questions to be asked before the interview focuses the need and helps the selection process. A job description should already have been written and should be discussed carefully with candidates. Candidates should be encouraged to ask questions regarding the job and the organization. They should have a clear understanding about the organization's philosophy and mission.

A great disservice is paid to both parties when a job is made out to be wonderful when it has a downside—and most jobs do! For instance, most HIV/AIDS programs work with individuals and families some of whom will eventually die. Employees need to be aware of this because they do become attached and losses are painful. Multiple losses are even more painful, and if they are not recognized and on-the-job grieving is not condoned, allowed, or supported, burnout can occur. Management makes a horrible mistake when everything that is said about the job is positive and the negatives are lost in the superlatives.

Team Interviewing

If the advertised job is in a team setting, it is invaluable to have two or three team members interview the candidate together. One member of the team should be of the same discipline as the prospective candidate and the others should represent other disciplines and departments. Before the interview, each interviewer should agree on the questions to be asked and who will ask what.

The advantages of this type of interview include giving employees a sense of responsibility toward the organization, other employees, and the candidate; having different personalities and disciplines represented provides a better overall picture of the candidate; the candidate has the opportunity to gain more in-depth knowledge of the organization; expectations on both sides are more likely to be met; if the candidate is hired there will be an increased commitment to the new employee's education and training; and the group's intuitive feeling helps in making the decision to either hire or not hire. The disadvantages are that it is time consuming and costly to get everyone together for the interview and it may cause stress to the candidate to have more than one interviewer. However, it is also an opportunity to see how the candidate handles that kind of stress, which is not a bad thing. HIV/AIDS organizations need people who can handle a lot of stress.

Skills

People can and do apply for jobs that do not match their abilities. Skills lists will find this out earlier rather than later. A skills list asks whether there is comfort in doing a procedure, when the skill was last performed, and whether a review or new training is necessary.

Secretaries and telephone operators should have their skills tested. Front-desk personnel can make or break organizations. Abrupt, brusque speaking voices and lack of understanding of the organizational mission and the client population can do more harm than is imaginable, as this person is usually the first and last contact a caller has with the agency and he or she may be speaking to a potential client who is already nervous and afraid.

Do remember that ancillary staff should be trained as well. A good answering service is an asset beyond price—a poor one is frustrating to would-be clients, clients, and staff alike.

Salaries and Benefits

Women in particular still seem to have difficulty in discussing money and benefits. Too often women appear not to think through their monetary value but rather to hold an attitude of "what do I need financially to survive." Employers and potential employees save themselves a lot of future hassles when they are clear about salaries, pay periods, overtime, compensatory time, vacation time, holidays, sick time, compassionate time, mileage, health options, dress codes, hours of employment, probationary periods, educational benefits, disability programs, pensions, savings plans, and any other benefits.

Interviewees need to be clear before the interview what they want financially, how much salary is livable, and if the job is worth the salary and benefits. For example, you are offered a job you can absolutely taste because it is what you really want to do. It is a 40-mile round trip from home and pays under $10 an hour with no increase in the foreseeable future. You are a single-parent head-of-household with three school-age children. This job will probably turn into a nightmare. Financial stress is a major stressor. It is important to be realistic and to think before you leap. This is important advice for you to give to clients.

After Hiring

New employees need to be recognized as just that. They need time to learn the faces and names of those around them and the whereabouts of personnel and supplies. Too often, understaffed and overstretched programs neglect this vital area of employment. There should be a structured orientation program and supportive supervision and evaluation for those who are providing direct care. Ideally, the new employee should be assigned a buddy who is there for them during the first few weeks to show them the ropes, answer questions, and monitor progress. Lack of support and training during this period can cause a new employee to resign in frustration and despair!

The End of the Probationary Period

If the new employee is not cutting it by the end of the probationary period, in most instances they should be advised of this and terminated. Too often, agencies do not do this for a variety of humanistic reasons. This is usually detrimental to everyone, and the consequences are rarely good. If the employee appears to be getting a grasp and is settling into the organization but is still dependent on training and supervisory support, then discuss this with the employee, be specific about his or her needs, and decide together on a date when a decision will be made to hire the individual permanently or to let him or her go.

STAFF RETENTION

Developing a reasonably stable and contented office needs understanding, humor, motivation, knowledge, conflict resolution skills, courtesy, ambition, loyalty, and good communications skills. Too often agencies seem to only manage by crisis. There is little long-range planning, and goals and objectives are changed with alarming regularity. The introduction of coherent policies with thoughtful decision making resulting in competent action is sacrificed to adrenaline-producing and energy-depleting waves of unfocused activity that may or may not avert the current situation and certainly do not foster growth or harmony. Every program will have crises, but when crises become the modus operandi they are not good news. This type of management behavior causes employees to want to stay in bed when the alarm rings, and they are heard to wail, "I don't know what's going on," "I'm always the last to know," "I just work here," "No one tells me anything," and so on.

Management by crisis can be changed through some simple strategies. A good place to start is with a weekly diary meeting for upper and middle managers.

Diary Meetings

A diary meeting is just what it sounds like. Every Monday, at a specific time, morning or early afternoon, the identified management personnel arrive and meet with the ED. Everyone has his or her diary or weekly calendar with them. A designated person takes minutes that are sent to each attendee by the following day. The previous week is reviewed. If there are things that need to be attended to, they should be addressed now. Each person then discusses his or her action plan for the week. The plan will have input from the ED and other members of the team.

A diary meeting has a number of things to commend it to managers. It provides a regular opportunity to review and maintain short- and long-term goals and objectives; it ensures immediate needs and tasks are resolved in a timely fashion; it prevents costly and frustrating duplication of services; it fosters checks and balances, self-monitoring, and accountability; it provides informal support and an opportunity to develop camaraderie; it encourages the resolution of conflict; and most valuable, it should ensure that all employees receive the same messages, free of hyperbole and jungle-drum gossip regarding the organization's needs, goals, and actions.

Conversely, American companies seem to hold an incredible number of meetings, starting at 7:00 A.M. with breakfast and going on, one after another, well into the night. The participant is numbed by the flow of words and exhausted by the continuing intellectual demand. Does this prolonged torture accomplish very much other than tired eyes, a weary body, and a desire to find a desert island and never leave?

Meetings

Getting the best out of meetings requires careful preplanning. Preplanning decides the goals and objectives and who should attend. A written agenda should be circulated to the attendees beforehand so that they can prepare for the meeting. A local oncologist insists that meetings start on time, minutes be taken, there be opportunity for discussion and feedback, consensus be reached, and specific tasks be assigned before adjourning. He believes that, with few exceptions, meetings never need to last longer than an hour. The results are productive, no one is exhausted, and all leave knowing what is expected of them and the time frame for the expectations to be accomplished.

Organizational Charts

Organizational charts are visual maps that clearly identify the organization's hierarchy. They show the governing body at the top with the ED immediately below. Similar to a family tree, there are solid horizontal and vertical lines that define the departments, departmental heads, and those who report to each departmental head. Broken lines depict those jobs or personnel who liaise with other departments.

The function of an organizational chart is to provide structure to all personnel regarding the size, departments, and reporting mechanisms of the company. Every employee should have easy access to the organizational chart so that there is no misunderstanding as to who is whom and who reports to whom, which, if not known, can become confusing, embarrassing, and stressful.

There are many small things that managers can do to instill and maintain motivation, loyalty, high individual esteem, and win–win situations.

The Successful Manager

This is the person who leads by consistent and continuous example. This individual knows organizational behaviors are established and maintained by the person who is at the top. Motivated, enthusiastic, and dedicated employees are those who are shown courtesy, respect, affirmation, and the ability to use their multiple talents in a growth-oriented environment.

Courtesy and Respect

Showing respect starts at the beginning of the workday. Do say "good morning" to each staff member. I once had a boss whose mood of the moment was judged by how she entered the front door. Her belligerent expression, nonverbal behavior, and short, hard steps were communicated faster than jungle drums through the office, and everyone made themselves as invisible as possible. Those whose main jobs were outside the office made fast getaways out the back door. The day was spent waiting for the proverbial other shoe to drop on some unfortunate victim, whom you fervently prayed would not be you. A day started with a smile and a friendly word sets the tone for the day. Sadly, too many businesses still seem to be run by fear rather than by motivation.

Criticism

Criticism should be handled behind closed doors. There is nothing more harmful than to abusively attack someone in front of his or her coworkers. It demoralizes everyone, gains negative comments, and rarely resolves a problem. Criticism should be given in private and phrased in a positive, clear and concise manner, and the employee should be invited to explain why the problem occurred. Both parties should participate in finding a sensible and timely resolution. If it is a serious infraction, a written report should be made, signed by both parties and placed in the individual's personnel file.

Saying "Thank You"

Agencies that work in the HIV/AIDS arena are constantly subjected to a variety of stressors. Workloads are frequently heavy, and individual accomplishments can be lost in the rush. Do remember to applaud tasks and deeds well done. Write a card, make a note on the annual evaluation, or develop an employee-of-the-month award that can be as easy as assigning a marked parking space, a mention in the office newsletter, or a gift certificate to a local mall. Be as objective as you can be. Some employees are a lot better at letting their good deeds be known than others. Remember that praise and thanks need to be appropriate or they lose their sincerity.

Don't Judge Others in Advance

Employees come in a variety of personalities, some of which we are instinctively attracted to more than others. This can mean that we jump to conclusions that can be false and give more praise and credit to those whom we like. Observation, listening, dropping our judgmental hang-ups, and keeping an open mind mean that all employees have a better opportunity of being treated fairly, which is all that anyone can ask and expect.

Timeliness and Details

Do know what is going on in your organization in every department. The health care motto is "If it is not written, it is not done." Office memos should be sent to all employees when there are policy and procedures changes, unscheduled meetings, office picnics, changes in security codes, changes in billing procedures, death in an employee's family, and so forth. The original memos should be kept by year in a three-ring looseleaf binder that is available for all employees to read.

Complaints

Complaints should be dealt with as soon as possible after they are reported. The people involved with the complaint should meet and investigate the complaint together. The complaint and the solution should be documented. The solution should be sent to whomever raised the complaint as soon as is feasible. If this is not immediately possible, let the person know what steps are being taken toward resolution.

Staff Support

Ninety percent of HIV/AIDS organizations are extremely supportive of their clients but are sometimes unresponsive to staff needs. Learning about stressors and being able to recognize their signs and symptoms helps to prevent employee burnout. Although the manager cannot and should not take on an employee's personal problems, nevertheless providing support is both humane and practical. Staff support can be offered in several ways, including listening and providing some objective feedback; encouraging them to rank their needs in importance and to tackle them one by one; suggesting solutions that, because of their own confusion, they may not have thought of; giving them one or two mental health days off to take care of needs, whether those needs are practical or emotional; prioritizing their workload and asking others to take over some of it temporarily; suggesting another area of employment within the organization; or suggesting that this may not be the workplace for them and that you would be willing to help them seek other employment.

Managers who acknowledge and assist stressed-out employees are rewarded by higher levels of teamwork, respect, and endeavor.

Projects

Bosses who always spend their off-duty hours dreaming up yet another new project remind me of those of us who find it irresistible to pass a walled construction site without looking through the cutout peephole! We vicariously enjoy watching others work. Some managers have the same mentality. The new project requires certain people to drop everything that they are doing and be assigned tasks for which they neither have the time, budget, personnel, and, because this is the same old repetitive story, the inclination, knowing that the boss will have forgotten the project in a few days or weeks. This is an appalling waste of personnel, who become frustrated, angry, hostile, and expect that it's only a matter of time before the whole cycle starts over again.

A new project should always be reviewed by the key department heads. If the project is considered worthwhile, an identification of responsibilities, assignation of tasks, and progress datelines should be agreed on, documented, and communicated to the responsible employees. Progress should be monitored regularly and challenges resolved before they become crises. The end result will be something that everyone is proud of, accomplished with a maximum of efficiency and a minimum of stressors.

Maximizing Individual Potential

Many of us work at our very best when we are well trained for the assigned job, are paid commensurate with our education and skills, are valued for our worth within the organization, believe in the organizational mission, and have the opportunity to continue to grow.

Growth invariably means change, and this is not for everyone. Those who do want growth should be encouraged to do so by enhancing their education, acquiring other skills, and continually upgrading their knowledge. So often new employees are hired externally, whereas if managers addressed the company's future needs and reviewed the skills and abilities of their current employees, jobs could often be filled from within.

Sharing Credit

Be generous in sharing credit. Staff usually hear all the negative things but are not always praised for their achievements. How frequently have we had a boss who claims that he or she is the inventor of every fresh idea when in reality these ideas come either from an individual or from a group of coworkers? Sincerely giving credit to whomever deserves it fosters goodwill, enhances your own stature, and provides a stable environment for people who are more than willing to be there for you when you need them.

Remember Your Own Worth

Sometimes employees forget just how much a good leader does for them. When this happens, there is absolutely no harm in gently reminding them of what you do for them. This causes the employee to pause and recognize the truth. It encourages them to rethink where they may have been coming from at a particular moment and to acknowledge you as a person of value and merit.

The work environment is by no means the responsibility of just management. Employees have an equal share in caring for themselves, understanding their own stressors, and intervening before these stressors become totally overwhelming.

INDIVIDUAL WORK-RELATED STRESS MANAGEMENT

Recognizing Personal Stress

How often have we seen stressors manifesting in others and remained resistant to the idea that it was happening within ourselves? For example, a social worker met with a counselor in her place of employment, surrounded by her team co-workers. For the past 2 years, her clients had been mothers and children with full-blown AIDS. She had had a lot of client losses to death, was frustrated by her own feelings of inadequacy, had little time for fun, and expressed an increasing sense of letting the team down. She spoke in short, terse statements: "I'm fine," "I'm OK," and "Leave me alone." At the "leave me alone," the tears poured down her cheeks while her face remained flat and remote. There was a long silence from her teammates sitting around the table, who seemed to communally hold their breath. She then said in a tone of bewildered surprise, "You know, I don't feel anything anymore." When quietly asked how long she had not had any feelings, she replied "Several months." Her tears eased somewhat, and she started to talk about her angers and resentments. The conversation began to involve other team members who were concerned and supportive. They were also frustrated because they said that they had recognized that her stressors were working overtime and had brought this to her attention but that she just hadn't believed them. The agency is very caring and extraordinarily compassionate. The help was there if she would have believed the staff messages. Sometimes our own denial gets in the way of our receiving help.

Learning our own stressors and recognizing our personal signs and symptoms are the keys to early diagnosis, intervention, and treatment. A warning sign for me is when I find myself silently swearing at aggressive and rude drivers weaving in and out of traffic on the overcrowded roads that usually do not bother me.

STRATEGIES FOR STRESS REDUCTION AT WORK

Support Systems

Support systems are those systems that work for us. For some, it is a nonjudgmental spouse, relative, peer, partner, or friend who is able to listen, sort out the reactive subjective stuff, feed it back to us, help restore a sense of equilibrium, and delineate possible options. No matter how desperate the situation may seem, there are almost always options, although they may not be visible if stress levels are high, clouding our objective vision. More formal help can come from an employee assistance program and regular support groups.

Employee Assistance Programs

These are administered by the organization's human resource department or contracted with an outside agency. They provide professional counseling in both personal and work-related issues.

Support Groups

A regular support group at work has much to commend it. It is held within work hours and should be available to all employees. There do need to be guidelines: The facilitator should be neither management nor an employee, confidentiality is sacrosanct, the support group should be for support and not a gripe session, it should not be mandatory, it should start and end on time, and a list of outside resources should be available for employees whose needs are greater than can be met by the group.

Support groups have several benefits if there is a high level of trust, communication, and confidentiality. Individuals can review their own beliefs and value systems while having the opportunity to understand those of other members of the group. Conflict can often be resolved by hearing another person's point of view. Perceptions are changed when one realizes that all jobs have their own stresses and strains. Even when some situations cannot be changed, if there is support from the group there is not such an "I'm-in-this-on-my-own" feeling. Groups fail when the facilitator and group members cannot overcome their own subjective feelings, allow confrontation, leak confidences to the boss, and cannot accept other group members' beliefs and values. This causes distrust, betrayal, anger, a sense of impotence, and helplessness—a failed group.

Well-run groups often have unseen positive results to the individual and the organization. When we feel included and our feelings are validated, our self-esteem is enhanced; we genuinely cooperate with each other and are more energetic and creative in reaching agency goals and objectives.

Other stressors are inflicted by the very nature of HIV/AIDS. It is a constantly progressing retrovirus about which new information is brought in on an almost daily basis. Clients often know more than the health professional who serves them. This can be discomfiting and stressful for both parties.

Maintaining and Enhancing Skills

To provide the best care, the health professional must be constantly aware of the ever-changing needs of those with the disease, the medications for prophylactic use and opportunistic infections, and the available social and financial resources. This is challenging for anyone. Do attend regular educational inservices, join the local community HIV/AIDS task force if there is one, attend conferences that are specific to your needs, and subscribe to an HIV/AIDS newsletter that provides up-to-date information in an easily readable format.

We all need support at some time. Don't be afraid to reach out and ask for it. In a caring organization it will be there for you.

Informal Office Support

Playing with people with whom you work is a great way to relieve tension, share a laugh, increase your social life, do some interoffice networking, and understand your coworkers a lot more. Having fun can include an inclusive "families-invited" agency picnic, smaller dinners with themes as simple as everyone wearing yellow or as novel as pairs coming dressed as book titles and everyone guessing the book, flying kites on the beach, a spiritual retreat (Kelly, 1995), or a night out to a casino. Having fun is as creative or as simple as you want to make it. All it needs is desire, enthusiasm, a little organizing, and participation.

Now that we have looked at taking care of ourselves in the work setting, let's look at life at home and how to manage this as well as possible.

Making the Most of Home

For many of us, the working day does not end when we leave our place of employment. We may have already worked 10–12 hours and return home to kids, pets, dirty dishes, untidy rooms, loaded laundry hampers, and a meal to be cooked. Our desire is to either collapse in a heap or escape to Tahiti!

Our personal lives are proceeding and have their own landmark events. Family births and deaths, children leaving school, mortgages to be paid, loans to be made, divorce, separation, abusive relationships, and neglected relationships all leave little time to see, let alone smell, the roses. Constantly neglecting our own needs eventually culminates in the production of unmanageable stressors. Those stressors affect our everyday lives at home and at work and may eventually lead to physical and emotional illnesses. This would not seem to be at all desirable. However, there may be some perceived kind of masochistic gain in always being miserable, exhausted, and martyred. If you don't wish to continue to be like this, it is useful to take a careful mental and written inventory of your current habits, behaviors, support systems, and concurrent life events to understand whether you need professional help now or can develop a personal plan of renewal that will start and keep you on a new and more fulfilling track.

STRATEGIES FOR STRESS REDUCTION AT HOME

Health Checkup

A health professional's task is to help clients look after their physical and emotional well-being. Sometimes we neglect to do the same thing for ourselves. Visiting the doctor is at the bottom of our priority list. We don't have the time, cannot afford it, think we are just fine, and so forth. We have to practice what we preach. Before embarking on any kind of stress reduction program, do go to your physician for a thorough checkup. Some of the stressor signs and symptoms may be caused by a physical condition. Physical problems should be looked after sooner rather than later. Discuss your work and home life with your physician. Ask for his or her suggestions on what lifestyle behaviors you need to change (you probably know already!) and how to go about doing this. For instance, weight training and aerobic exercise may be contraindicated at this time because of a physical condition.

If you don't like your present physician, shop around for a new one. Find one who takes the time to discuss his or her findings with you, address your concerns, and recognize the type of work that you do. Find one who is younger than you so that you are both not retiring at the same time! As part of your good health campaign, see your physician at least once a year, and more frequently if you notice bodily changes.

Professional Help

If you are completely exhausted, constantly tearful, feeling emotionally empty and abandoned, losing weight, picking fights with whoever crosses your path, can't get on with anyone at work, feeling you are a total failure, criticizing everyone, having little concentration, cannot sleep at night, having an increasing need for chemical substances, and driving recklessly, put down this book and make an appointment with a counselor immediately.

If, however, you have some of the above signs and symptoms but they are not presently interfering noticeably with work or at home, do something about them before they get out of hand and intervention and treatment are no longer optional.

One of the most visible signs of increasing stress is a pattern of sleep interruptions and disturbances.

Sleep Disturbances

Sleep disturbances can be caused by difficulty in falling asleep, nightmares, restlessness, leg cramps, prolonged periods of wakefulness, asthma, allergies, common colds, and assorted aches and pains.

Our lifestyles affect our ability to enjoy a healthy, restful sleep that allows us to awake refreshed to tackle the challenges of a new day. Behaviors that interrupt good sleep patterns include regularly using prescription and over-the-counter sleeping medications (they are a temporary fix and may be habit forming); the overuse of alcohol, which acts as both a stimulant and a depressant; the use of illegal drugs; heavy cigarette smoking; overeating, particularly of fatty foods; drinking caffeinated beverages in the afternoon and evening; taking naps during the day; fighting with family members; going to bed angry; watching murder and mayhem on late-night television; untreated aches and pains; the day of the week (many sleep better on the weekends); and refusing to let go of the day.

Do remember that sleep is a very individual function. Some of us need more or less sleep than others. Most people do well on 7½ hours, but this is just a general rule.

Sleep is helped by avoiding sleeping pills as a permanent solution; cutting down on alcohol and smoking; reducing the intake of caffeine at night, including chocolate; exercising in the early evening; taking 15 minutes for yourself to unwind; soaking in a bubble or herb bath; avoiding stressful tasks before bedtime, such as paying bills or cleaning closets; keeping a notebook by the bed and writing in it rather than lying awake restlessly; getting up and drinking a mug of warm milk or caffeine-free chocolate; practicing relaxing all your muscles by lying on your back in bed and alternately tensing and relaxing each set of muscles, starting with your feet and working upwards until you have reached your face (do this several times until you can feel the tension leave your body and the relaxation seep in); avoiding watching or reading violent television programs, films, or books before sleep; avoiding stressful telephone calls unless it is an emergency; investing in a comfortable mattress and pillows; listening to meditation tapes; and then enjoying a good night with sweet dreams and waking revitalized in the morning.

Exercise

How many excuses we make not to exercise! How many of you have a stationary bike, exercise step, or a Jane Fonda tape tucked away where the eye cannot see it and the conscience cannot mumble over it?

Exercise is without a doubt emotionally and physically enhancing. Just getting out of the house or apartment and strolling around the block can change our perceptions, lift our spirits, and improve our well-being. The hardest part is leaving the couch! Regular moderately vigorous exercise, three to four times a week for 20– minutes, will increase cardiac output, strengthen flabby muscles, and increase endurance. Regular exercise includes walking, jogging, running, aerobic conditioning, swimming, dancing, in-line skating, bicycling, tennis, handball, squash, and weight training. New studies among people over the age of 60 have shown that muscle strength can be substantially increased through supervised weight training.

Before beginning any exercise regimen, check it out with your doctor. When you start, don't try to become fit in your first week. Be kind to dormant muscles and carefully monitor your progress. Do warm-up and cool-down exercises before and after each session.

If exercising on your own takes too much effort, ask your partner or a good friend to commit to joining you at certain times during the week. Signing up with a gym is also motivating as you throw money away if you don't use the facilities.

Many hospitals and communities have supervised wellness programs that charge very little, are age related, and are held at various times of the day and evening to fit all schedules. Do remember that exercise should be fun; most of us are not training for a marathon!

Overeating

Many of us handle stress by eating comfort foods. Chocolate chip cookies, rum raisin ice cream, corn chips, pretzels, peanuts—the list can go on forever, as can the weight! We watch the scale slowly reflect our transgressions and bargain that we will take it off when "I'm 10 pounds/20 pounds/30 pounds overweight." In the meantime, our cholesterol is probably increasing at the same time as our waistlines!

Too many of our children have adult role models who introduce them to junk food, candies, calorie-laden desserts, and cookies as a way of life and not an occasional treat. These habits become a part of our adult lifestyles. If you are a compulsive overeater and heavily overweight, the easiest way to overcome this (and it's not easy!) is to join some kind of weight-reduction plan. Research this with your physician. Many of the programs are not cheap as you not only sign up but agree to buy their products. Obesity is extremely unhealthy; the only cure is to change the behaviors and attitudes that you hold toward eating. The average snacker can usually take charge of his or her eating habits by learning what is meant by a nutritious diet. Nutrients include the following.

Protein. Protein maintains and builds body tissues, manufactures hemoglobin, and builds antibodies to protect us from infection.

Vitamins and food supplements. Most physicians contend that if we eat a balanced diet, we do not need vitamin supplements.

Minerals. At the least we need calcium (dairy foods), iron (beef and fortified cereals), phosphorous (dairy foods, meat, fish, poultry), iodine (seafood, iodized salt, milk), magnesium (legumes, seafood, nuts, green vegetables), zinc (meat, seafood, cereals), and copper (seafood, meat, cereals, nuts, and raisins).

Fat. Yes, we do need fat, but not nearly as much as most people eat. Fat is classified as saturated, mono-unsaturated, and polyunsaturated. Fat should make up no more than 30% of our daily intake of calories. Nowadays as food labeling has improved, we can read the labels and purchase food products accordingly. There are now fat-free milk, sour cream, yogurt, cookies, cakes, and cheese and all sorts of reduced-fat items. We need to read before we buy.

Carbohydrates. Carbohydrates supply energy and fiber to the body. Simple carbohydrates are sugar based; complex carbohydrates are the starches and soluble and insoluble fibers.

Water. Water is the principal component of blood. It carries away the body's waste and regulates our body temperature. Water is cheap, clean (one hopes), refreshing, and necessary.

Menus

Shopping will be quicker if you make out a week's list of menus and buy accordingly.

Shopping

The art of grocery shopping is to make a list and stick with it. This means that you do not fall prey to advertising gimmicks, shelf placement of high-priced low-content foods, and other blandishments. You will also save money, which is a definite plus. Shop on a full stomach, and shop when you have the time and if possible when the supermarket is not busy, which is usually early and mid-morning or later in the evening. Avoid shopping on the weekends; it can be a zoo.

Reading Material

Purchase a pocket-sized fat gram counter. *The Low Fat Supermarket Shopper's Guide* has broken down "thousands of brand name foods and has come up with specific recommendations for fat content in all product categories" (Katahn & Pope-Cordle, 1993, p. 3). This little book provides an extraordinary amount of information and quite a lot of surprises about one's favorite comfort foods! *The 8 Week Cholesterol Cure* (Kowalski, 1990) is also very useful. It is an easy-to-read guide to lowering cholesterol levels without too much hardship.

Thinking Thin

Choose the amount of weight that you want to lose and set a realistic time frame in which to lose it. Weigh yourself once a week only, at the same time, and on the same scale. Obsessing with the scale does not help, so stay off it between times.

Imagine yourself the size that you want to be. Do this whenever you want that extra candy bar, and think how great it is going to be to fit into the latest "with-it" swim gear you saw in the department store last week. Remember that there are going to be weddings, parties, and other celebrations to attend. The occasional pig-out will not hurt too much. As you change your eating ways, you will find that you will eat less and you actually don't enjoy your old eating habits. Don't talk food with friends. The vision of a large chocolate sundae may be just too much temptation.

Giving away the clothes that no longer fit may seem a little radical, but psychologically it tells us that we don't need them any more and that we are progressing toward our goal. Do give yourself a gift as you lose weight, for example, a pair of shoes, a scarf, a book, or a massage—something that reminds you of what you are accomplishing.

The more responsibility that you take for your own body, the better you will feel about yourself and about other people.

Taking Time

Each of us needs to regularly renew and replenish our bodies, minds, and spirits. So often, in the hectic pace of life that most people lead, the self is neglected. Enough neglect will cause emotional and physical disturbances.

Taking time for your needs should fit your personality and lifestyle. I take 15 minutes every morning to sit on the patio, read a thought for the day, think about the words in the writing, and allow myself to center so that I can actually feel the peace that is within. Even if there is apparent chaos in my life, I find that doing this is calming, stabilizing, and uplifting. When I don't do this, my day never feels as whole.

Taking time can mean telephoning a supportive, nonjudgmental friend and exploring life; keeping a journal or diary; putting your feet up and having a nap; walking on the beach; getting up really early and going to the local park to see the sun rise and hear the birds sing; taking up a hobby that has always appealed to you; returning to school to learn something new and unrelated to work; growing a garden; having a bird feeder that you can see from your window; shopping at the mall; reading a book that you have never had the time to; or getting a massage. The list can go on and on, but it is useless unless we choose to activate it.

Positive Thinking

I do believe that how we think affects our lives. Somehow those people who expect the worst always seem to have bad things happen to them. We all have challenges in our lives. The going will sometimes be extraordinarily rough, and all the positive thinking in the world will not alter events. How we think about them at that time and later makes the difference between growth and stagnation, hope and paralyzing fear, enthusiasm and negativity.

At a superficial level, negative thinking means that we will never find a parking space, we always join the wrong line, and the bank will close just before we arrive. Deeper negative thinking dampens our enthusiasm for life, decreases our ability to set and achieve goals, keeps us in the same old rut because we are terrified of change, and prevents us from living a happy and fulfilled life. A happy and fulfilled life does not happen by itself. We need to desire it, be willing to work toward it, and recognize that it is a lifetime goal and that responsibility for its achievement is ours.

Self-Worth

"Positive thinking is the belief in our own self-worth, and in the value of everyone else. That belief leads to self-confidence, respect for others and a life-style based on strong values" (Fellman & Peale, 1995, p. 1).

Developing Self-Confidence

To do this, we need to explore our own values and beliefs. Fellman and Peale (1995) have stated that there are seven master values that make up the chief principles in people's lives: honesty, courage, enthusiasm, service, faith, hope, and love.

It's up to you to analyze how you feel, interpret, and behave toward these master values. Most of us have had times when honesty may not seem the best policy, we have embroidered the truth, or we have felt singularly devoid of faith and hope. Discussing these values with family and friends will make for a lively conversation and an insightful revelation. When we enhance our values by living by them as a code of ethical conduct and belief, we open the doors to opportunity and change.

Opportunity

There is not one of us who has not had opportunities that we have foregone either for valid reasons or because of absolute fear—fear of the unknown, fear of losing everything, fear of change. Years ago, I fell in love. The love lived in another country, and so one of us had to move. We were both at the peak of our careers, enjoyed our jobs, were making our mark, and had a lot of support from friends, family, and our respective communities. Eventually, after much soul searching, nail biting, and kicking and screaming, I was the one who moved. I said to my spiritual advisor, "What happens if it doesn't work—I have burned all my bridges." She said calmly, "So what? Just start again." Talk about returning me to basics. Well, it worked wonderfully. Indeed, there were a lot of roller coaster rides, but we went forward with faith, hope, and enthusiasm, and our love and commitment to each other has strengthened through 17 marvelous years.

Seizing opportunities means taking a large step over a precipice. The parachute is made up of self-worth, beliefs, hope, ability, risk-taking resourcefulness, and the spirit of adventure. Seizing opportunities means that we do not have to live our lives with if-onlys. Once the first step is taken, other opportunities seem to unfold in front of one.

Finding the Good

Every day we are pounded by the media with all the horrible things that people do to each other, animals, and the environment. In the office we are all too quick to point a finger at someone else, gossip about each other, and share somebody else's secret. We can choose to listen, read, and watch upbeat information; we can refuse to participate in maligning someone else; and we should always keep someone else's secret. We were privileged to receive it and should treat it as such.

Establishing Goals

For life to have purpose and meaning, it needs to have goals. Goals should not just be long range. The more that we learn to live our life in the here and now rather than in yesterday or tomorrow, the more contented we will be. Working with people with HIV/AIDS should be a strong and poignant reminder that life does not last forever and that we should make the most of what we have today.

Goals are different for each one of us and should not be cast in concrete as they do change along life's way. Making them gives us a blueprint for action. Short-term goals could include learning a foreign language, developing an always-wanted skill, enjoying a long weekend break nearby but not at home, becoming computer literate, or going back to school. Long-term goals could include traveling to exotic places, spending more time with family, improving financial stability, and volunteering for a local HIV/AIDS organization or a worthwhile program totally different from your work environment. Giving back to others is profoundly rewarding. You always receive more than you give. Goals are individual but won't be accomplished if we keep on saying "I'll do it next year."

Procrastination

It's extremely easy to become so bogged down in the events of each day that we constantly make excuses as to why we cannot do the things that we believe would enhance our lives. Maybe they won't, but we won't know that until we try. We say "I'm already too busy/tired/broke/not in the mood/overwhelmed; I cannot possibly do one more thing." Try—just for a week! Early each morning, make a list of the things that you have to do each day. Then prioritize them from 1 to 10 and do them, starting with Number 1.

Don't put off tasks that you don't like. They don't go away and will have to be done, and the deadline for them could change. Regard them as a challenge and tackle them with that upbeat attitude. Don't put off the task because it has to be perfect. It may never get done. Look at your goal list, decide where you want to start, and act on it today.

Have a major office and home cleanup. Time is wasted looking for things, and it's truly amazing how much junk we collect. Uncluttering our environment helps to unclutter our minds. Either have a yard sale or pass items on to a thrift store. Your junk may be someone else's treasure.

Keep a written timetable of how you spend your time. Include refreshment breaks, telephone calls, office interruptions, meetings, and appointments. At the end of each day, assess your time use and decide whether you could have used it more efficiently. For instance, would it be easier to return your routine telephone calls in a block at the end of each day? This may not be feasible, but then again it may be.

Eat your lunch away from your desk. Taking a break refreshes the mind and improves the afternoon. Sign up for a time management class. They do work and provide insight into how and when time is wasted. Maintain a calendar or diary that clearly shows all of your appointments with an address and contact telephone number.

No chapter on stress would be complete without mentioning self-guided imagery, visualization, massage therapy, music therapy, and art therapy. All of them increase our awareness, decrease our anxiety and paranoia, and improve our well-being. Find which works for you and do it regularly.

CONCLUSION

This chapter has addressed stress and stressors and has suggested what causes us to move into a place of disequilibrium and why. It has looked at stress in the workplace and at home and has offered a number of suggestions on how to efficiently manage stress.

Ultimately, individuals must be able to assess their own stressors and choose to take those steps that will either relieve or reduce them to everyday challenges rather than overwhelming afflictions.

REFERENCES

Antonovsky, A. (1979). *Health, stress and coping.* San Francisco: Jossey-Bass.

Blattner, B. (1981). *Holistic nursing.* Englewood Cliffs, NJ: Prentice-Hall.

Fellman, E., & Peale, R. S. (1995, March 15). The power of positive thinking, 1995. *Bottom Line Personal, 16,* 1–2.

Friedman, M., & Rosenman, R. H. (1974). *Type A behavior and your heart.* Greenwich, CT: Fawcett.

Guralnik, D. B. (Ed.). (1976). *New world dictionary of American language* (2nd ed.). Cleveland, OH: The World Publishing Co.

James, J. (1987). *Windows.* New York: Newmarket Press.

Katahn, M., & Pope-Cordle, J. (1993). *The low-fat supermarket shoppers guide.* New York: W. W. Norton.

Kelly, J. (1995, April). Please do not disturb. *Travel and Leisure,* 58–63.

Kowalski, R. (1990). *The 8 week cholesterol cure* (Rev. ed.). New York: Harper & Row.

Maslow, A. (1954). *Motivation and personality.* New York: Harper & Row.

Rando, T. A. (1984). *Grief, dying and death.* Champaign, IL: Research Press.

Vachon, M. L. S. (1987). *Occupational stress in the care of the critically ill, the dying, and the bereaved.* Washington, DC: Hemisphere.

11

Where We Are
and Where We Are Going

We have learned, of course, a lot about the disease since 1983. We know perhaps less about the disease itself, which is still mysterious. And we don't know how to treat patients. —Luc Montagnier (1994), The Pasteur Institute

In 1995, HIV/AIDS continues to be a mystery. As one research discovery is made, another challenge arises and has to be unraveled. The virus is remarkably adaptable and mutates regularly. Continuing research and effective treatment and care will continue to be needed until a preventive vaccine and a curative medication can be found. Research has made many strides, but still has a long way to go before HIV/AIDS becomes a distant unwelcome memory of yesteryear.

RESEARCH

Identification of the Virus

For years, there was a long-standing dispute as to whether Dr. Robert Gallo at the National Institutes of Health (NIH) had "used a sample from the French virus to create the American version of the tests for the human immunodeficiency virus (HIV) which causes AIDS" (Herman, 1994, p. 10). A concession was made by NIH in 1994 that stated "that American researchers used a virus obtained from French competitors" (Weiss, 1994, pp. A1, A11). This has enabled the renegotiation of the original contract of 1987 between NIH and the Pasteur Institute, which now gives the Pasteur Institute a greater share of the royalties from the French and American test kits. Luc Montagnier, the French virologist whose team first isolated the AIDS virus, said "it's the end of a bad story" (Herman, 1994, p. 10). This story is told to remind us that many people and countries worldwide are researching HIV/AIDS issues and that those who discover an efficacious vaccine or a cure will be heroes in their own country and in the rest of the world.

Vaccines

According to a report compiled by the National Institute of Allergy and Infectious Diseases (NIAID),

> *a growing number and variety of experimental vaccines are entering clinical tests in primates and humans, and more trials are exploring whether changing immunization schedules, increasing booster doses or using a combination vaccine strategy can stimulate stronger, more durable immune responses. (NIAID, 1994)*

Researchers at the Harvard AIDS Institute have reported in the journal *Science* that "infection with the second, milder, AIDS virus, HIV-2, sharply reduces the chances of becoming infected with HIV-1, the virus causing the AIDS epidemic. These findings suggest a new avenue for research . . . and delivering it in the form of a safe vaccine" (*The Weekly Telegraph*, 1995).

Another vaccine is also under research, according to NIAID. An article written by the Associated Press (1995) reported that "researchers think the most effective AIDS vaccine is likely to be a live virus, which will prime the body to mount a spirited reaction to HIV" (p. A3). Many, though, worry about giving healthy people even a weakened form of the AIDS virus because it might cause cancer, immune suppression, or even AIDS. Because of these fears, a team from NIAID is developing a live but weakened virus that can be killed off once it does its job. Although a lot more testing is necessary, it is yet another approach that just might work. The World Health Organization (Associated Press, 1994) has said that "heterosexual male drug users in Thailand and homosexual men in Brazil will be the volunteers of the first major human tests of two AIDS vaccines" (p. A22). The tests are planned to begin within the next 2 years. They are intended to be performed in a large-scale study of between 3,000 and 20,000 people. This is very positive news, and one hopes the results will be equally positive.

Life Spans

According to a 1994 article in the *New York Times* ("HIV Patients Living Longer," 1994), a study in San Francisco has found that people infected with the virus are living a year longer than they were in 1983. There is a small group of Australians who were infected by blood from a single donor, all of whom seroconverted and have remained healthy. Several hundred people infected with the AIDS virus have remained healthy for more than a decade. The reasons for this are under intensive study, but in the meantime good health should be maintained for as long as possible through medical intervention, a healthy lifestyle, and a positive attitude.

Women and Children

Traditionally, women, children, and minorities have been left out of research studies. For years, all diseases were studied in White males, and although the medical community began to study female, childhood, and minority illnesses in the 1980s, it would seem that HIV/AIDS has given a powerful impetus to providing money for more adequate research in this very needy population. One only has to see the effects of giving zidovudine (AZT) during pregnancy (chapter 3) to applaud these efforts and hope that they will continue.

Medications

One of the reasons that people are living longer is that the clinical treatment of the opportunistic infections is better understood and more effective. The antiviral drug AZT is still suggested as a prophylactic intervention for those patients whose T4 cell counts fall below 500, but research has shown that although survival seems to improve rapidly among first-year patients, Dr. Jens Lundgren of Hidoure Hospital in Copenhagen found that "patients who survived more than two years while taking AZT had a higher death rate than untreated patients" ("HIV Patients Living Longer," 1994, p. A17).

The antiviral drugs ddC, ddI and d4T are now approved by the Federal Drug Administration. The drug ddC was approved to be used "for those who can no longer take AZT either because they have developed resistance to AZT, or because they experience severe side effects from AZT treatment" (Van Heertum, 1994, p.31). Multidrug combination therapy has become increasingly popular, both prophylactically and for opportunistic infections.

Many of the medications have severe and uncomfortable side effects. Clients should never be coerced onto any medication protocol. They should fully understand how long it will last, what the hoped-for outcomes are, what possible reactions there can be, how frequently the medication is taken, the route by which the medication is administered, and if there is a 24-hour "comfort" telephone number to call for support and to have questions answered before the protocol is begun.

Many areas of the country now have research sites, very often through community research initiatives. Do find out if there is one in your area and what they have to offer.

Research has a long way to go, but it is the vital link to the prevention and cure of HIV/AIDS. No matter how much research is done, nothing will stop the present exploding global population of HIV/AIDS-infected individuals.

THE WORLD

Much of the world has believed that HIV/AIDS would not affect their country. Subsequently, nations are not prepared to provide education, diagnosis, or treatment interventions. Furthermore, some of the countries that are, or will be, hardest hit are those that are the poorest and whose women have traditionally held the role of second-class citizens. These women have had little choice in either their sexual partner or their medical care. In 1994, "by conservative estimates, there [were] now 17 million people infected with HIV worldwide, three million more than a year ago" (Brown, 1995, p. 5).

Many times, advocacy and awareness has come from individuals who have taken it on themselves to do something. There is the wonderful story of Tekie Gebie Mariam who walked 750 miles from Addis Adaba, the capital of Ethiopia.

He is a 64-year-old grandfather whose mission was to talk to as many people as possible about HIV/AIDS and sexually transmitted diseases (STDs). His primary targets were the young people of Ethiopia. A nongovernmental organization in India is promoting that explicit and fascinating manual on sex, the *Kama Sutra*, to say "that sex with one partner in many positions is safer than sex in one position with many partners" ("Indian NGO Features *Kama Sutra* in Safe Sex Campaign," 1993, p. 7).

Luc Montagnier claimed that the "disease has stabilized, and is even declining in parts of northern Europe" (*The Weekly Telegraph*, 1995). If this proves to be true, it is extremely good news. However, there is real concern that the general population in northern Europe will hear this message and stop listening to the educational information regarding prevention, transmission, and spread, a Catch-22 situation!

The "have" countries must begin or continue to cooperatively and creatively assist the "have-not" countries in finding and funding economical ways to promote safe sexual behaviors; socially market cheap, safe, easily available condoms; develop peer education programs, clinics for STDs, and HIV testing, diagnosis, treatment and care; adequately train clinic physicians and staff; develop alternative or complementary approaches to the prevention of the spread of HIV by injecting drug users, such as needle-exchange and bleach distribution programs; clean up and deliver a safe blood and tissue supply; and develop partner notification systems.

THE UNITED STATES

According to the 1994 year-end edition of the Centers for Disease Control and Prevention's (CDC's) *HIV/AIDS Surveillance Report* (1995), 80,691 cases of AIDS were reported in 1994. Although this was a drop from the 1993 figures, the number was "substantially higher than the number reported in 1992 which was 47,572" (p. 5). The AIDS epidemic is still primarily affecting men who have sex with men. The same report stated that "men represented 82 percent of AIDS cases reported among adults/adolescents 13 years old or older" (p. 5). Young men aged 20–24 were particularly at risk. Of those who were reported to be HIV-infected, 60% reported having sex with other men. These figures would indicate that prevention messages are not getting through to younger gay men, and that effective risk reduction strategies must consider the current social and psychological issues rather than using the prevention and educational themes of previous years.

This report (CDC, 1995) also indicated that we need to address where AIDS educational dollars are going. For years, the gay community raised its own funds and developed its own educational programs. Now that there is money available, the gay community should not be left out. According to an article in the *Washington Post* (Hamilton, 1994),

a survey by the Institute for Health Policy Studies at University College of San Francisco found that while gay males represented 77 percent of all AIDS cases in California, only 7 percent of those served by state funded programs are homosexual. In contrast 18 percent of those served by state programs were heterosexuals at risk, even though

trast 18 percent of those served by state programs were heterosexuals at risk, even
though heterosexuals represent only 2 percent of the AIDS cases here. (p. A6)

If one looked at the nation as a whole, there would probably be found a similar allocation of funds. The same *Washington Post* article stated that "a recent survey found that one third of gay and bisexual men in San Francisco between 17 and 23 reported having unprotected anal sex in the previous six months" (p. A6).

Young gay males are in many ways no different than their heterosexual counterparts. Their hormones are active, they feel invincible, and they cannot believe that safer sex is the only way to go. Where they differ is that they may be unable to "come out" because of familial, cultural, and social taboos and are therefore afraid to seek education that specifically talks to gay men.

Pedro Zamora, an outspoken activist from Miami who died in 1995, said at a World AIDS Day speech in 1993, "I ask you to think about the reality of an adolescent who has never learned about condoms from a health teacher who is straight, and who has heard nothing but shameful messages about being attracted to other men." Older gay men find it difficult to relate to this younger generation. They have nursed their sick, changed their behaviors, come out, reached frequently into their wallets, and may feel that they have done enough. Education and intervention must be developed before this generation repeats the history of years past.

Education for Gay or Bisexual Men

The most effective education seems to be taught by peers. Although it must include safer behaviors as a permanent life change, it also needs to address the issues of a positive self-image and self-esteem; negotiation and assertiveness; erotic alternatives to intercourse; cultural and ethnic values and beliefs; outreach to gay bars, restaurants, and churches; and ongoing support groups.

It is also known that older gay and bisexual men have relapsed in safer sex behaviors (Jones, 1994b). Again, there has to be a long-term commitment to adequate educational funding if behaviors are to change and stay changed. Both the Gay Men's Health Crisis in New York and the AIDS Resource Center in Dallas have recognized this challenge and have developed relapse-specific intervention programs called, respectively, "Keep it Up" and "Keeping it Up." It is essential that these programs are adapted and adopted throughout the country if the gains made among gay and bisexual men in the 1980s are not to be lost in the 1990s.

Women and Children

For several years after the discovery of HIV disease in America, the impact on U.S. women was in no way similar to their sub-Saharan counterparts, where women had been and continue to be infected at similar rates to men. That pattern has dramatically changed, and the proportion of cases among women has increased steadily during the past decade. During 1994, AIDS among women represented 18% of adult and adolescent cases (CDC, 1995). This report found that most women were infected either through injecting drugs or by heterosexual contact with an infected man. Most women reported with AIDS were Black or Hispanic (57% and

20%, respectively). The infection among children increased 8% over the previous year, and 92% of these cases were transmitted perinatally. There is a disproportionate impact of the epidemic on minority communities, where it is 6 or 3 times higher, respectively, among Blacks and Hispanics than among Whites.

Education for women and children. This vulnerable population still does not always believe that it is at risk. Educational messages must be delivered in ways that are culturally, ethnically, socially, and economically understandable. Education needs to be ongoing, condoms need to be of good quality but inexpensive and available, and negotiation skills and assertiveness training must be key educational elements in preventing the further transmission and spread among women, adolescents, and children..

Often there is distrust of the medical system because of past experiences, particularly among Black and Hispanic populations. A study conducted by Johns Hopkins University "shows that Afro-Americans do not seek care, do not receive it, and often fail to have the risks of HIV adequately explained. They are also less likely than their white counterparts to receive [*Pneumocystis carinii* pneumonia] prophylaxis or anti-retroviral therapy before visiting an HIV treatment center" (Chavez, 1995, p. 17).

The reasons for this are multiple. Effective education must understand the underlying causes of mistrust and previous systemic inequities before it will be able to communicate life-saving messages.

Affected children. Affected children are those whose parents and siblings are infected with HIV/AIDS and who face the prospect of losing everything that is their known world. They need to have their future lives assured, where possible with their own input; this will let them know that they will not be left alone or abandoned when the parent is either ill or dies. Although this brings up all sorts of tough questions to be answered and determinations to be made, most children will do better when their fears are addressed truthfully and they are aware of what their future holds.

Children should be treated as children; they need to shout and laugh and play. A dreadful disservice is done to them, however, when they perceive that they are excluded from events and decisions that will affect the rest of their lives.

Counselors need to be remarkably sensitive to everyone's needs and wishes. Through family counseling, they can help the family reach a consensus of agreement that will help the children to survive well.

Counselors also must recognize that many families will have "family secrets." Secrets are those hidden things that no one ever mentions. They include illegitimate children; alcoholism; physical, emotional, sexual, and economic abuse; child and elder abuse; criminal behavior; incarcerated relatives; prostitution; pimping; or the possession and use of illegal drugs and the selling of illegal drugs. Injecting drug users are particularly at risk for the transmission and spread of HIV/AIDS, and it would seem pertinent at least to consider them.

NEEDLE-EXCHANGE PROGRAMS

There are needle-exchange programs in existence. However, a variety of restrictions and barriers have limited the number of programs, and currently fewer than 50 exist nationwide.

Restrictions and Barriers

Most states have laws that ban the distribution of syringes and needles and require a prescription to obtain them. Negative public attitudes have helped politicians to avoid changing these laws. There is also a ban on the use of federal funds to carry out needle-exchange programs (Jones, 1994a). There are some (illegal) underground programs to which the community turns a blind eye, but that attitude can change without notice.

An Existing Program

Baltimore, under the leadership of Mayor Kurt Schmoke and at the instigation and relentless lobbying of its Health Department, was eventually able to change Maryland state law to entitle the City of Baltimore to establish a pilot needle-exchange program. Changing the law took several years. It required the enormous effort of contacting not only legislators but community programs, health organizations, and religious and business groups. The rationale behind the program was carefully explained as well as the intention to tie HIV education to drug treatment whenever possible. Baltimore is to be congratulated for its commitment and stamina to succeed.

Costs

Needles and syringes are a lot cheaper than the annual cost of treating an adult or child who is HIV-infected. Furthermore, if people can at the same time be encouraged into drug and medical treatment, the humane aspects cannot be underestimated.

The positive and negative effects of needle-exchange programs in this country will not be seen for several years. It is hoped that they will be positive and will encourage other communities to develop similar programs.

Over the past 15 years, funding for HIV/AIDS has moved from absolutely nothing to a myriad of financial assistance.

FUNDING

Funding is now available through federal, state, and sometimes local governments. Ryan White funds have made an enormous difference to infected and affected communities and are available in most major cities. They can be used for a variety of interventions. The Medicaid AIDS waiver has assisted infected individuals in staying at home rather than in an acute care institution by using case management and delivering contracted services within the home. Social Security has made it easier and quicker for infected individuals to claim benefits, even though the paperwork can still be distracting.

Private foundations have donated enormous amounts of money to affected cities, some from very early on. Three that immediately come to mind are the Robert Woods Johnson Foundation, the American Foundation for AIDS Research, and the National Community AIDS Partnership, begun by the Ford Foundation. Their extraordinary, prolonged, and continuing contribution can never be overestimated.

WORLD AIDS DAY

World AIDS Day is December 1. Each year, more and more communities around the world find a way to publicize, educate, and fund-raise for the HIV/AIDS epidemic. It is also a time when candlelight vigils are held, the Names Project panels are displayed, and those who have died are lovingly remembered. Make certain that your community uses this day to promote AIDS awareness, particularly in schools, churches, and synagogues, and to commemorate the lives of those who have died.

A 5K run/walk has been held in Ft. Lauderdale for several years. This event is fun and has become known as a major fund-raiser for HIV/AIDS needs. The money raised is distributed by a grant process available to all types of HIV/AIDS direct care organizations. The distribution is divided equally between education and direct care. The run/walk finishes with a candlelight vigil in a park by the river. To be a part of several thousand loving people is a beautiful and moving experience.

CONCLUSION

As this book was written, every day, throughout the world, more people—men, women, and children—became infected with HIV. We have yet to find a vaccine or a cure, but progress is being made.

The people who appear to live the longest would seem to be those who have chosen to change their risky lifestyles, eat healthily, exercise regularly, find their spiritual pathway, remain involved members of the community, surround themselves with positive support systems, and know how to use community resources. They are the people who like to take as much control as they can and make their own decisions regarding care and treatment after listening and weighing all of their options. This is not possible for everyone. Care and treatment is often expensive, distrusted, and far away.

Women cannot easily change the cultural and social mores that support men having sex with other women or with other men.

The cumulative total of AIDS-related deaths in the United States now exceeds 300,000. Worldwide, the virus appears to be set to explode in high-risk population such as injecting-drug users, children and adolescents sold into the sex trade, and those infected with untreated STDs. Those infected will in turn infect others unless education can make itself an integral and effective part of society.

The health professional can actively assist in this country, and in other countries, to proactively counsel affected and infected persons. Counseling should support, advocate, and intervene in an ethical, consistent, and compassionate fashion. HIV/AIDS is scary, and it does result in many losses. We can make a difference to our clients by being there for them and by providing avenues of practical, emotional, physical, psychosocial, and spiritual caring that will enable them to face their multiple challenges with hope and not despair.

REFERENCES

Associated Press. (1994, December 17). First Major AIDS vaccine test for Thailand. *The Sun-Sentinel*, p. A22.

Associated Press. (1995, February 1). "Timebomb" AIDS vaccine promising. *The Sun-Sentinel*, p. A3.

Brown, P. (1995, January). HIV: The story so far. *Panos World AIDS, 37*, 5–8.

Centers for Disease Control & Prevention. (1995). *HIV/AIDS surveillance report: Year-end edition 1994*. Washington, DC: U.S. Department of Health & Human Services.

Chavez, L. (1995, March/April). Pride, prejudice and the plague. *Positively Aware*, 16–19.

Goodman, W. (1994, April 12). Television reviews: AIDS research: The story so far. *The New York Times*, p. 24.

Hamilton, W. (1994, August 24). In San Francisco, grim AIDS cycle poised for encore. *The Washington Post*, pp. A1, A6.

Herman, R. (1994, August 2). French scientist focuses his AIDS research. *The Washington Post*, p. 10.

HIV patients living longer. (1994, April 13). *The New York Times*, p. A17.

Indian NGO features *Kama Sutra* in safe sex campaign. (1993). *Global AIDS News*, 4.

Jones, P.M. (Ed.). (1994a). Initiating needle exchange programs. *AIDS Information Exchange, 11*(3).

Jones, P.M. (Ed.). (1994b). Safer-sex relapse. *AIDS Information Exchange, 11*(4), 1–7.

National Institute of Allergy and Infectious Diseases. (1994). *NIAID background: HIV/AIDS vaccines*. Washington, DC: Author.

Van Heertum, A. (1994, August 12). Anti-HIV drug approved. *The Washington Blade*, p. 31.

Weiss, R. (1994, July 12). U.S. concession settles HIV dispute. *The Washington Post*, pp. A1, A11.

Appendix: Resources

The following HIV resource telephone numbers are very useful. They are usually manned by volunteers who are friendly, knowledgeable, and helpful.

AIDS National Interfaith Network	(202) 546-0807
American Indian AIDS Institute	(415) 626-7639
American Life Resources Corporation	1-800-633-0407
CDC National AIDS Hotline	1-800-342-2437
	1-800-344-7432 (Spanish access)
	1-800-243-7889 (TTY, deaf access)
	1-800-AIDS-101 (Creole access)
Choice in Dying	1-800-989-WILL
Drug Abuse Hotline	1-800-662-4357
Hemophilia and AIDS/HIV Network for Dissemination of Information	1-800-424-2634
LAMBDA Legal Defense and Education Fund, New York City	(212) 944-9488
Medicare	1-800-366-7586 (Mon.–Sat., 8:30 a.m.–5:00 p.m.)
National AIDS Clearinghouse	1-800-358-9295
National Association of People with AIDS	(202) 898-0414
National Clinical Trials Information Service	1-800-874-2572
National Minority AIDS Council	(202) 544-1076
National Pediatric HIV Resource Center	1-800-362-0071
National Women's Health Network	(202) 347-1140
Pediatric & Pregnancy AIDS Hotline	(212) 430-3333
Social Security Administration	1-800-772-1213 (7:00 a.m.–7:00 p.m.)
Teens Teaching AIDS Prevention Program National Hotline	1-800-234-8336
The Orphan Project	(212) 925-5290
United States Railroad Retirement Board	(305) 356-7372

Index

ACLFs (adult congregate living facilities), 88
Acquired immunodeficiency syndrome (AIDS) (*see* HIV spectrum disease)
Adolescents, risky behavior of, 16
Adoption, 49–51
Adult congregate living facilities (ACLFs), 88
Advance directives, 97
Advertisements, 5–6
Advocacy, 2–3, 57–58
AFDC (Aid to Families with Dependent Children), 84–85
Affirmation, 144
Affirmative prayer, 111–112
Africa, 73
Aid to Families with Dependent Children (AFDC), 84–85
AIDS (*see* HIV spectrum disease)
AIDS National Interfaith Network (ANIN), 108
Alcohol rehabilitation programs, 17, 37
Allergic reactions, to spermicide, 39
Americans with Disabilities Act (ADA), 65–66
Anger, 110, 134
ANIN (AIDS National Interfaith Network), 108
Anonymity, 65
Anticipatory grief, 14–16
Art therapy, 54–55
Asia, 6–7, 73
Attorney, for deceased, 125, 126
Attorney-in-fact, 66–67
Audiocassettes, for children, 55
Awareness stages, of HIV-infected children, 56
AZT (zidovudine), 8, 26, 35–35, 177

Banks, 126–127
Behavior
    in grieving, 135–136
    risky, 16–17
Belief systems, personal, 153
Benefits, 128–130
Bereavement
    activities during, 143
    groups, 144–146
    concurrent life events, grief recovery and, 133–134
    importance of, 115
    intervention, for children, 147
    rites/rituals, 122–123, 138–139, 147–148
    sexual relationship during, 142–143
    specialists, 131
    (*See also* Grief)
Bereavement Support Group for Children, 147
Birth certificate, adoption and, 50
Bisexual men, 3, 5, 179
Black Americans, 41, 92, 179–180
Blame, 139
Blood circulation, with approaching death, 117
Blood transfusion recipients, 17
Blood-borne transmission, 14, 17
Body disposition, options for, 123–125
Burial, 124
Burnout, 150, 155

Cambodia, 6
Camps, for HIV-infected children, 55
Carbohydrates, 168
Caribbean countries, 6
Case management, 83